DANCING WITH CANCER

A HEALING THROUGH

VISUALIZATION

DANCING with CANCER

A HEALING THROUGH

VISUALIZATION

Robert E. Elliott, Ph.D.

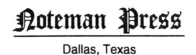

Noteman Press

Dallas, Texas

01-651

ISBN 1-886597-01-4

Library of Congress Catalog Number: 94-69908

First Printing, December 1994
Second Printing, June 1997

Printed in the United States of America

Cover Design by Jeff Boswell

NOTEMAN PRESS
2603 Andrea Lane
Dallas, Texas, 75228

214/327-4466

CONTENTS

Multiple Myeloma
Information
"Indolent" Myeloma
Treatment
Secrecy
Feelings
Group 17
The Fall into Terror
The Thousand-Dollar-a-Minute Machine
Psychotherapy
Inward Journey
The Powerful Female
Killing Cells
"Brute"
Brute in Group 17
Brute at Work
Where are the Healthy Cells?
Diana
Achterberg and Lawlis
Achterberg and Lawlis II
Couple Therapy
Hera and Diana
The Dance

FOREWORD

Bob Elliott presented himself to my office on his own referral in the spring of 1991. He had been diagnosed in 1980 with a plasma cell dyscrasia, very often an early harbinger of a bone marrow malignancy called multiple myeloma. He had been followed appropriately without treatment by another oncologist for many years, since his disease process seemed to be relatively indolent. By 1991, however, laboratory testing reflected a more malignant growth of his disease process. Oral chemotherapy had been recommended, and the patient wanted a second opinion. I had met Bob on several occasions at some of the psychological seminars that were held in the local Dallas area. Bob apparently wanted an oncologist who was somewhat more flexible in his approach to psychological affects on disease processes. Because Bob wanted as minimal side effects as possible, including hair loss, so that he could continue practicing as a psychotherapist, we agreed on a relatively mild oral chemotherapy regiment. For more than three and a half years the patient's multiple myeloma has stayed under excellent control, and indeed has shown improvement of his disease process during this period of treatment.

A significant segment of the general populace loves to embrace the stereotypic, pure logic, no-nonsense physi-

cian who is unwilling to accept any suggestion of the potential benefits of non-conventional therapies, particularly those in the psychological realms. A favored saying
in medical school was "if it can't be scientifically proven
in a prospective, randomized, double-blind, statistically
analyzed study, it's not true." Bob knew that I had a foot
both in the scientific world as well as the world of psychological healing. Bob was not one of those unrealistic people who wanted to choose between medicine versus psychological tools to get better. He preferred the more reasonable route of "using every club in the golf bag."
Throughout the entire course of the patient's treatment, he
has made me aware of his different, in depth, psychological healing maneuvers. This book is Bob's personal story
about "travel into unchartered territory."

Bob's rich imagery about his disease process and the
imagery that he utilized as a form of psychological treatment always has been fascinating and intriguing. I can
remember as a medical student often being fascinated with
the stories about the "Type A" personality in heart attacks.
It always made sense to me that tiny and subtle molecular
changes throughout the body, generated by stress, could
certainly have an adverse affect on the cardiovascular
system, with the ultimate result of a heart attack twenty or
thirty years down the line. I am not so convinced that
those same minute physiologic changes can result in the
destruction of a malignant tissue process. I perceive the
"hard-wired" genetic changes associated with cancerous

growth and the "software" input from psychological resources are not evenly matched.

I was particularly impressed with Bob's description of his relationship with his wife, which reaffirmed my belief that "relationships are the stage where we all work out our issues." I think Bob summed it up well when he stated about the book that perhaps it could be "an encouragement and stimulus to a reader to explore some of his own pathways to self-discovery and self-healing."

If one believes in an after-life experience, and thus presumes there is a purpose for our existence on this earth, I am of the belief it is to learn something. In one book on after-life experiences, the author made the statement that no matter which culture one reads about near-death experiences, a common theme seems to be that people had a sense that they were asked two questions as they glimpsed "the other side:"

(1) Did you gain in wisdom?

(2) Did you learn to love?

If that is our quest in this existence, then I would suggest that Bob Elliott has come a long way in "doing his homework well."

One of the more interesting aspects of Bob's journey was his very interesting graphing in chapter *Three* of his blood proteins, which have reflected the activity of his disease process correlated with his vivid imagery. Being realistic, it would be impossible to determine how to separate out how much of his disease process was affected by the chemotherapy and how much was affected by his psychological energies. I do appreciate his correlation of the "cell-killing Brute" with "cell-killing chemotherapy" on the one hand, and the Dancer with biological response modifiers on the other. In his imagery the Dancer transforms cancer cells back into healthy and beautiful white cells. The parallel between that drama and the ability of biological response modifiers/cytokines to alter the genetic response of cancer cells is certainly intriguing.

Perhaps my favorite part of Bob's book is his statement that "the story validates itself." Maybe life is about dancing, and those who learn the dance will not only enjoy it more but may even live longer.

Robert W. Burns, M.D.

PREFACE

I first met Bob in 1968 when I accepted a faculty position at Perkins School of Theology, Southern Methodist University. He had preceded me there by a dozen years, as he had in the graduate program at the Divinity School, University of Chicago, of which we both are alumni. After nearly a decade as colleagues at Perkins, I preceded him into private practice by a couple of years. Then we were office mates and friends until I disrupted our daily association by marrying Helen Hunt and moving to New York. That move merely decreased the time we spent in contact, but not our comradeship and trust.

That trust was expressed by Bob's making me among the first who knew that he had cancer. What I remember most about that meeting was his calm demeanor and the absence of emotional devastation. That was not surpising in retrospect, since he had already survived a previous diagnosis some eleven years earlier, and had had open heart surgery after that. It was not his style to take things passively, but with active curiosity and hope. Ever since I had known him he was an inveterate workshop attendee, constantly curious about his personal dynamics, always optimistic and creative. And immensely intelligent.

The other honor Bob bestowed on me was his invitation to read the early versions of this manuscript and to offer any suggestions I might have. The drafts have gotten longer and better despite my advice. As time has passed, Bob has become clearer about what he thinks about his experience of staring the dark intruder in the face, proficient in delaying his encounter with the afterlife, and more philosophical, which accounts for the lyrical quality of this essay.

This narrative is not only a journey of Bob's probing the mystery of his blood cells "acting out." It is an equally fascinating journey through the minds of other explorers of the mind/body boundary. In the process of his self study and self treatment and his education in the literature, he has become an expert witness. He has included stories and studies of fellow travelers who have experienced the mystery of our complexity, of the human commitment to survival in the face of unspeakable odds, and a person's ability to influence the functions of the blood cells with images, hope, courage and endurance.

Most important to me is the evidence of the deepening awareness in the field that a supportive community, while no guarantee of immortality, is essential in the delaying the grim reaper. Bob, although modest in his claims to do so, offers genuine hope and guidance for other travelers on this perilous journey.

I read the book with tears in my eyes that one of my best friends was threatened with a too early death, and with admiration that he would not go gently into that dark night. I feel great appreciation for deepened hope and illumination I have received from Bob and his fellow travelers. I am relieved that the manuscript is finished and that he is not. In fact, to me he seems more alive and feisty than ever. He'll probably reach the new human life span of 120 years, and die with a smile on his face. No matter what or when it happens, Bob has learned to dance, and with his dance we all revel in the vibrancy of full aliveness. Hurray Bob!

Harville Hendrix, Ph.D.
Abiquiu, New Mexico
November 1, 1994

(Dr. Hendrix is author of *Getting the Love You Want* and *Keeping the Love You Find*, best-selling guides for couples and singles.)

ACKNOWLEDGMENTS

This book tells a personal story that reveals much about me. As you will discover, it is also about my wife Dorothy, our relationship and our marriage. Thus to her, first of all, goes my gratitude for her willingness to allow this story to be told in this way. My love, respect and gratitude for her partnership with me in this journey are beyond any simple saying, and should become clear in the telling of the story.

Somebody has said that when the student is ready the teacher will appear. Somehow the right teachers have appeared for me along the path of my journey and I want to acknowledge and thank them here:

First of all, thanks go to my psychotherapist Jean Johnson. You will read how she was present at the beginning of the imagery journey and served as a wise and skillful guide through all but the most recent parts of it.

Jeanne Achterberg and Frank Lawlis appeared at the right time to help me through a difficult stuck place in the journey. Other wise friends who showed up in timely fashion with the right comment or the right question to facilitate the next step in my journey include Rosalind Frank, Donald Weaver, John Shaffer and Tom Simpson.

Of those who helped "prepare the way" by nurturing my growth as a person and therapist, above all come

Joseph Zinker and members of therapy Group 17. As you
will discover, they play a major part in this story. Other
guides on the imagery journey in ways more helpful than
they are likely to know are David Grove, Martin Rossman
and David Bresler.

Then comes a long list of personal friends with
whom I have shared accounts of my journey in progress,
and who have consistently and patiently and lovingly sup-
ported and encouraged me in this journey and in my
writing about it. I owe special thanks here to Harville
Hendrix, Gay Jurgens, Fred Stovall, James Hall, William H.
Farmer, Fred Seipp, Cathy Bingman, Joyce Tepley, Don and
Ruth Lamka, Phil and Phoebe Anderson, Carole Carsey,
Dave and Margie McKeon, Susan Ellis, Francine Daner,
Rick Spletter, Gayle Wilson, David Switzer.

Not least on this list come our daughter Marla Beth
Elliott and her husband Dan Rader, our son John, and son
Bruce and his wife Victoria. Their loving and appreciative
response to this story has meant a great deal to me.

My oncologist, Robert Burns, has been a good friend
as well as a good doctor. He has always been honest and
straightforward with me about what he knows, what he
does not know, and about what he thinks. He often doesn't
know what to think about aspects of my psychological
journey (sometimes I don't either); but he has consistently
welcomed my trying to find ways to play an active part in
the treatment game. I am fortunate to have found him.

My thanks to a wise, gentle but incisive editor, Lucille Enix, who has saved this manuscript from clumsy constructions, unclear sentences and numerous other infelicities.

As my first words of appreciation go to Dorothy for her loving company on this journey of healing, so here my final words of thanks go to her for her good company in the task of writing. Her tactful, wise and practical suggestions have helped make the text more coherent and readable. Readers should be grateful. I am.

INTRODUCTION

"Depend upon it, sir, when a man knows he is to be hanged in a fortnight, it concentrates his mind wonderfully."

- - - Dr. Johnson

The sentence of execution came for me in 1980 in the form of a diagnosis of multiple myeloma, a rare blood cancer described in the medical literature as incurable. Though I knew even then that I had much longer than two weeks before the execution, I had no idea how far in the future it lay.

As it turns out, I have negotiated a stay of execution for more than fourteen years and, as of this writing (late 1994), seem to have the cancer in retreat.

The sentence was announced twice, in 1980 and then again in 1991. For ten years after the first diagnosis, my myeloma lay dormant, or, as the doctors say, "indolent," not calling for treatment. After my initial scared reaction, I allowed the myeloma to retreat from the center of my attention, but it remained like a small dark cloud on the back horizon of my mind. Something was there, but maybe the diagnosis was wrong.

No such luck. In early 1991, the small cloud suddenly erupted into a terrifying black thunderhead. The myeloma was on the move. Blood tests showed aggressive advance, and I began a regimen of chemotherapy to combat it.

I also took seriously my responsibility to participate with the doctor in my own treatment. I began a journey of self-discovery and self-healing that has taken me to surprising places and remarkable outcomes. The following pages tell of that journey.

I have learned to wrestle with this cancer and, even more astonishingly, to *dance* with it, in a way that seems to transform its terrible energy into something creative and life-giving. That claim may sound rash, but in the following narrative I will try to make it at least plausible.

I realize that I was able to come to this journey, this struggle with cancer, with some valuable psychological and spiritual resources. As a practicing professional psychotherapist and former seminary professor of pastoral counseling, I have learned to value "inwardness," to trust the process of inner exploration, and to be open to a loving wisdom greater (or deeper) than my conscious mind.

Few of my readers will share that precise background. Some will share parts of it. But I trust that what I have written will strike some chord of deep recognition in most readers.

The heart of this book is the narrative of a personal inward journey, employing a process called visualization or imagery. As I made my way inward in search of ways to cope with this deadly cancer, I was astonished to encounter images that raised again profound personal issues I thought I had long ago worked through and resolved. These issues had to do with an archetypal, powerful and dangerous female *(anima)* image in my psyche. Apparently I had not finished with that work after all because I was now being challenged to struggle again with it. That struggle has taken some unexpected turns and opened into some surprising new discoveries and transformations, of the cancer, my life, and my marriage.

Although I have tried to weave this story into a coherent sequential narrative, variations in style will reveal that it has been put together from segments written at different periods during the last two years. Some portions sound impassioned, frightened, even angry, others more contemplative and calm. Some parts share intense personal experiences from "inside," others offer a more objective and detached look at research information about cancer. There may even be some inconsistencies---as my views of some matters have shifted in the course of my journey.

For recall of events in that journey I have depended on journal notes made at the time, conversations of recall with friends who had roles in the story, and on my own memory. For some of these events memory is misty, but for others it is as vivid as if happening only yesterday.

My psychological and spiritual journey effectively began in the spring of 1991 with the activation of the dormant cancer, and the beginning of chemotherapy. That inward journey continues to this day and is not yet finished. But it has brought me to a place I think fitting to share with readers in the hope they may find it interesting and helpful.

ONE

MY JOURNEY

"Maybe what's most deeply
personal is also what is most
truly universal."

---Carl Rogers[1]

Multiple Myeloma

I began chemotherapy for multiple myeloma in the spring of 1991. This rare form of blood cancer had first shown up in my system eleven years earlier. In 1980 my internist had spotted a worrisome blip in a routine blood test (bless him for being so alert) and referred me to an oncologist, who made the diagnosis by bone marrow aspiration. This is a procedure in which some bone marrow is drawn out through a hollow needle tapped into the hip area of the pelvis. At that time, the myeloma seemed to be at a very early stage, so the oncologist recommended that we watch it carefully but not yet begin treatment.

The diagnosis frightened me. My wife and three grown children were also frightened, and together we had a couple of family therapy sessions to help us talk about this dark cloud over us all. Dorothy and I did several things to try to help me. We changed my diet in a Pritikin direction. (This was before the American Cancer Society was ready to recognize any link between diet and cancer.) We planned ways to reduce my work stress. I undertook some internal imagery work, following the lead of the Simontons in their book *Getting Well Again*.[2] For reasons I think I understand better now than I did then, the process did not prove very useful to me at the time. As you will discover, imagery work has come back into my life more recently in a dramatic and powerful way.

Information

I read as much as I could find about multiple myeloma. Since the disease is rare, the literature is not extensive.[3] Myeloma represents about one percent of all malignancies, about fifteen percent of all blood cancers.[4] I learned that the disease affects the white blood cells that are generated along with red cells in the bone marrow. Because white cells are major players in the immune system, the progression of the disease eventually compromises the immune system, leaving the body susceptible to infections and other diseases. In that way and some others it resembles AIDS. As the cancer cells multiply in the bone marrow, they also crowd out other healthy white cells and red cells, and in time penetrate the bone wall itself with tumors that weaken its structure. For most patients the first diagnosis occurs when the disease has already progressed enough to produce bone pain or bone fracture. I was lucky in being able to catch it early.

Multiple myeloma has no known cause and no known cure. It is considered incurable, though not untreatable. Doctors don't know of any myeloma patient who has not in time died of the disease (unless something else gets the patient first), but its course can be extremely variable. About half of all patients respond to treatment and half don't.

"Indolent" Myeloma

This disease has the interesting property of sometimes lying doggo for long periods of time. The medical terms for that feature are "indolent" or "smoldering." In my case the "indolent" period lasted eleven years. After the initial diagnosis, we followed it carefully with blood exams at frequent intervals. What shows up in the blood are not the cancer cells as such, which remain in the bone marrow, but certain proteins and other factors generated by the cancer cells. These provide an indirect but fairly accurate measure of the cancer activity.

When these markers did not advance but stayed steady month after month, and then year after year, my anxiety about the myeloma abated, and I found it easier to accept my internist's hope that we were looking at a benign condition that sometimes imitates myeloma.

That more placid state of affairs came to an abrupt end in February of 1991 when a routine blood test during my annual physical exam showed a marked jump in the protein level. Another visit to the oncologist, another bone marrow aspiration, and confirmation that my "indolent" myeloma was now waking up.

Bemused by that term "indolent," I wrote to a friend about that time:

"It's as if I had this lazy good-for-nothing son-of-a-bitch lying around on the back porch, swigging corn whiskey and swatting flies---no good to anybody but not much harm either. Now he has roused up and is stomping around in the garden, scaring the hell out of me. I'm trying to get him to lie down and be lazy again."

That is one image I cobbled up consciously and deliberately. Other images and metaphors I will be telling you about arrived more spontaneously and from realms more mysterious.

Treatment

It was now time to begin chemotherapy. A standard protocol for myeloma in early stages calls for low intensity dosage, administered orally for five consecutive days at intervals of about four weeks. We are currently using cytoxan (related to mustard gas) and prednisone, a form of cortisone which appears to have some kind of anti-cancer effect.

I worried at first that the chemotherapy would be debilitating, but that has turned out not to be true. All the way through since early 1991, I have been able to continue my work and other activities, including golf, mostly without disruption. Although we have stepped up the dosage considerably (450 to 500 mg. of cytoxan and 100 mg. of prednisone daily for five days), I have continued to tolerate it well. Indeed, the prednisone serves as something of an "upper," giving me an extra shot of energy during those days. That in turn creates something of a "withdrawal" problem: when I come off the meds, I have to taper down the prednisone so as not to drop in a depressive hole for a couple of days.

In the first few months, the doctor and I tried some different medications including vincristine, administered intravenously. That treatment had the unhappy effect of producing some nerve impairment in the form of numbness at my thumb tips, and to a lesser extent finger tips. My sense of balance also became more shaky and my hair began to thin.

As we switched back to the oral medication, these malign side effects abated. My numb thumb tips still make sorting papers a clumsy chore, and my wobbly balance has taught me to be very careful on even a short ladder. The numbness bothers me less, and it is hard to tell if nerves are repairing or if I am learning to adapt better. However, if my life or work required me to stand on one leg I'd be in big trouble.

The hair loss unnerved me and I made some inquiries about a wig, though I could not imagine any wig being successful at deception. Anyone familiar with my appearance would surely not be fooled, and my "cover" would surely be blown. Fortunately, the fall-out has abated, and I have not had to face that problem. My hair and beard have become much whiter, but that passes without much public notice.

Secrecy

After each of the two diagnoses, in 1980 and in 1991, I made the decision to keep the information about my cancer secret from all but my family and a few close friends. Motives for that were probably mixed. As long as I could function responsibly in my professional life, it seemed unnecessary and probably detrimental to have it known in the community and among current and potential clients that I have this serious disease. Cancer is a scary word that sets loose strange spooks in many minds, including my own. I know about that from memory of trying to minister to cancer patients as a young Methodist pastor.

By now, as you can tell from reading this, I have decided to reverse that secrecy decision---to come out into the open. Motives for that reversal are also probably mixed. They certainly include the hope that my work and my story may prove useful to other cancer patients and to those who work with them. It is my earnest hope that I may be able to make some of the things I have learned accessible to others.

Some of my long-time friends who read this will be surprised, and some may even feel hurt that this heavy secret was kept from them until now. It wasn't easy to know how to share it. Early on, when I was shaken and scared, I didn't want to cry on everybody's shoulder, though it was very important to have some specific shoulders to cry on. Later, as my imagery work began to unfold, and I became more encouraged about what was happening, it simply got too complicated to describe in any simple way:

"By the way, I have multiple myeloma."

"Gosh, tell me about it."

"Well, it will take me about forty minutes to tell you."

Not an easy conversation starter

Feelings

With the new diagnosis in 1991, I was flooded for a time with heavy waves of sadness and fear. After the visit to the oncologist, Dorothy and I sat on the couch and held each other and wept. A few days later I sat in my office leading a therapy group of people I had come to know and cherish over a long period of time. Something like grief filled my chest and squeezed my heart. It was as if I were already having to say goodbye to these people I loved.

That sadness eased after a while and has come to be replaced by a more exuberant sense of gratitude for the miracle of life, about which I will have more to say later.

About fear: that same year, I had the awesome experience of being held and supported as I plunged all the way, I think, to the bottom of my terror. It happened in Group 17.

Group 17

This is an extraordinary therapy group in which I have been a member for more than twenty years. Its history goes back to the 1960's, when members of the young Southwest Group Psychotherapy Society formed a training group. They invited a training therapist from New York, Cornelius Beaukencamp,[5] to meet with them periodically. As the group transmuted into a therapy group, Beaukencamp named it "Group 17," and it has kept that name through several changes.

The original members, many of them major figures in the group psychotherapy movement in the Southwest, have all cycled out and been replaced. The leadership of the group has also changed. For more than twenty years, it has been in the remarkable hands of Joseph Zinker, formerly Director of the Gestalt Institute of Cleveland, and author of *The Creative Process in Gestalt Therapy.*[6]

To describe here how Joseph and the members of this group have, over the years, nurtured, challenged, supported, chivvied, confronted and loved me into whatever manhood and maturity I can claim for myself would require another whole book. Here I will just tell you how they journeyed with me into my terror about the return of my cancer. In recent months I have come more often to look back on this experience as a pivotal event in my pilgrimage, so I want to try to describe it as carefully as I can.

The Fall Into Terror

This meeting was in early March of 1991, soon after the new ominous signal in the blood profile, and before the second bone marrow aspiration. My mood was apprehensive about an uncertain future. But I wanted the group to hear that I was calm and prepared to face bravely whatever might come. Sitting next to me was a dear friend who has herself had much acquaintance with physical illness and suffering. She kept gently and persistently pushing through my words in loving search of what was behind them. My calmness did not ring true to her and she wasn't going to let me get away with it. I am unable to recall much content of that conversation, but it peeled away more and more of what proved to be denial rather than real courage. My fear became more audible and palpable. They could hear it and I could hear it. I could feel it. It seemed to be about helplessness. I remember asking her, in a voice beginning to choke, "What can I do?"

Gravely she replied, "I don't know what to tell you to do, but I can tell you that I love you." My eyes closed and tears poured forth. As best I can describe the experience of the next few moments, I think I went down into a place of absolute helplessness and vulnerability. I was exposed and utterly naked. I didn't have a thing to hold to or to cover myself with.

Amazingly, it was all right to be there. It was as if I had gone all the way to the bottom of whatever this terror was and found that I could survive. I didn't explode, or implode, or blow away, or melt, or burn up, or any of those terminal terrors that attend our fear of finally letting go. I have heard clients say things like: "If I ever let myself begin to cry, I would never be able to stop" or, "If I ever let my anger out, it would be like a volcano destroying everything within range" or, "If I don't hold myself together real tight, I will disintegrate into a thousand pieces."

I don't remember which of these terrors was the most vivid for me. What I do remember is that I was willing, or able, or compelled (in some sense all three) to let go and to take the drop. Amazingly I found I could just be there. "There" had no tangible features, no furniture, no geography. Whatever "bottom" means, it wasn't even something to stand on. It was suspension in emptiness.

I also knew that this was happening before the eyes of my friends in the group. I was absolutely exposed before them, as helpless and vulnerable as a newborn. I must have trusted them---without such trust I could not have gone through this---to be there with me in my helplessness.

And they were there---quietly, gently, attentively. They didn't run away; they didn't get nervous; and they didn't try to "fix" me. Whatever their feelings, they didn't try to talk me out of mine. They didn't try to reassure that it wasn't that bad, that things would turn out well---any of the conventional "comforts" we are tempted to offer people in extremity. They were willing to be "there" with me in my "there-ness," and it was a profound gift for which I am deeply grateful.

Another perspective on this experience will appear on page 106 with the poignant account of the illness and lonely death of another multiple myeloma patient, a Catholic priest. For whatever reasons, he was unable to allow himself to enter that space of vulnerability, help-lessness and dependence on loving friends.

The Thousand-Dollar-A-Minute Machine

Sitting in the circle of Group 17, after a time (who knows how long?) I became aware that my hands were being held gently by the two women seated on either side of me. I blinked open my eyes and began to look around. Joseph began to speak. He asked the other group members to link hands, and asked me to be aware of the energy of love and healing flowing in that circle, flowing through me. As I looked around I could see as well as feel that pulse of loving energy.

Again, I don't remember how long that power circle was at work, but I know it to be one of the deep healing ex-periences of my life. Later, quipping partly to cover the remnant of my self-consciousness, I said, "Wow! If that circle were a machine I could get hooked up to in the doc-tor's office, it would cost a thousand dollars a minute!"

In later meetings with Group 17 I have mentioned the thousand-dollar-a-minute machine and how I might want to connect to it again. But, interestingly, I have not felt the need for it since then. It is as if at the crucial moment I was able to go where I needed to go, to do what I needed to do (not knowing until I got there what it was), and the group was ready and able to be there with me.

It seems to me quite likely that sometime in the future I may again have need of that thousand-dollar-a-minute machine, and it is comforting to know that it will be there for me to hook up to.

Psychotherapy

In addition to Group 17, I had the good fortune to have a good personal therapist at hand. Jean Johnson and I had been introduced to each other by a mutual friend who thought we might be interested in learning some things from each other. That turned out to be true. Jean is a gifted Neuro-Linguistic Programming teacher and therapist, and I have experience and credentials in marriage and family therapy. We hit it off well, and set up a schedule to trade off some teaching and consultation.

That process was just nicely under way when the roof fell in on me. "I want to change the contract," I told Jean. "I want your help in dealing with this death sentence I have been handed."

In the first couple of sessions, my way of talking about my illness must have sounded fatalistic or resigned, because Jean came up with a question that shook me: "Do you have a right to live?" I wrestled with it. I wasn't willing to say "No," but "Yes" didn't sound right either.

To say, "No, I don't have the right to live," sounded condemnatory, as if I were passing judgment on myself for some unspeakable crime.

On the other hand, it didn't sound right to reverse that and say, "Yes, I do have a right to live." That sounded pretentious, or self-righteous, as if I had a right to be an exception, a right to be granted a miracle, a right to be exempted from the natural processes that affect other victims of this "terminal" illness. What right did I have to claim such special status?

I couldn't put the question down and I couldn't answer it. I gnawed on it like a dog with a bone, with Jean egging me on.

Resolution, and immense relief, came with a slight shift in the wording of the question. As long as the question about my right to live implied, or seemed to me to imply, my right to be given something, I couldn't make either "Yes" or "No" fit. But when I shifted the question to: "Do I have a right to *do* something that may not have been done before?" the answer came easily. "Yes, I do have that right." I have a right to be a pioneer, to travel in uncharted territory. Maybe I can find something there that hasn't been found before. That is permission I do have.

The shift to "pioneering" released me from the impasse, and opened up the work I will now describe.

(When I told my daughter of my relief and pleasure at finding the idea of the pioneer, she sent me a little plastic model of Daniel Boone in a coonskin cap. I keep him on my office desk.)

Inward Journey

Imagine, now, my sitting in Jean's office, ready to work---if I can figure out how to work. How do I attack this mysterious invisible cancer that is threatening my life? Jean made a suggestion: "Why don't you take an imaginary journey down inside your bone marrow, look around, and see what you can find?"

Here begins the dramatic part of this story---an internal journey of remarkable discovery, involving visualization or imagery. If as a reader you find those terms unfamiliar, you may want to detour to Appendix B, where I have tried to provide some general description and rationale for this kind of process. Or you may choose to take a deep breath and plunge in with me here.

Because I had used visualization before and in work with clients, I was able readily to respond to Jean's invitation. In my mind's eye I miniaturized myself, as it were (remember Raquel Welch in the movie "Fantastic Voyage"?), and I soon found myself inside my bone marrow, looking around.

I didn't have to wait. Immediately I was confronted by a host of large, bulbous, soft, white, papery, balloon-like figures---half floating, half bouncing---coming at me in great numbers. Though slightly larger than I, they were light and easy to push aside or push back. They were also easy to puncture and deflate, so they had no apparent way of hurting me. Nevertheless, though I couldn't make out their danger to me, I began immediately to have the most uncanny, spooky, creepy, scared feeling.

"I don't like it here," I said to Jean. "I want to get out of here." However, because I had learned from past experiences that feelings like that are usually a clue to something important trying to get through to me, I also said, "I'd better hang in a while, to see what this is about."

It didn't take long. It suddenly came to me that these white bulbous figures were *female forms!* Later it occurred to me that they resembled the Venus of Willendorf, that famous prehistoric fertility symbol, faceless and limbless, all breasts, belly and buttocks. In my imagery, these figures were papery and soft, rather than made of stone, but they certainly were female forms.

"My God, Jean," I said. "Here is the story of my life: coping with the powerful, overwhelming female. Why is that now being acted out in my bone marrow?"

The Powerful Female

Time for some personal history: I grew up the oldest of three sons in a family with an intense, passionate, frequently angry mother, and a quiet passive father. By the time I had become an adult, and could look back on all that, I realized that my mother's anger was mostly at my father ---at his avoidance and passivity, his inability or unwillingness to meet her force with his force. He would retreat from her anger, which would fuel more frustration and anger in her.

A consequence was that a lot of her anger spilled over on me, and I frequently felt the target of anger I didn't understand and didn't know how to deflect. I tried to please her, but had little confidence in my ability to do that. So I learned to keep a low profile to try to avoid offending her. Now I realize that I came into adulthood with a bone-deep assumption, hardly conscious till years later, that women are powerful and "right," and men are not powerful and "not right." A somewhat wobbly platform for marriage.

You will not be surprised to learn, if you know how these things work,[7] that I fell in love with and married, in Dorothy, a woman strong, warm, and passionate, who turned out in time to have a great capacity for anger. The anger didn't show at first. But the stresses of a new baby with feeding problems, plus life in a new Methodist parsonage, began to press on both of us. Under stress I tended to revert to the low profile, avoidant pattern I had learned from my father. Dorothy began to feel abandoned, an old issue for her, and would let me know about it in a voice that carried more pain and anger. As her anger rose, I tended to retreat in dismay or to try to placate her, which generally made it worse. This pattern made for a lot of pain for both of us over a lot of years; at that time neither of us knew how to change it.

To oversimplify a long and complicated history, Dorothy and I developed a relationship that had much love and life in it, but one that got out of balance in serious and painful ways, including the realm of parenting. Following my father's example, I left much of the responsibility for family leadership to Dorothy, but would let her know subtly, and sometimes not so subtly, when I didn't like her decisions.

In many ways I set Dorothy up to be angry. Then I would retreat from her anger as if wounded, would sulk, get depressed, or---worst of all---try to act "nice."

It was Group 17 that really got to me on this one. Early in my history with that group, they pointed out after hearing a lot of my complaints, that it sounded as if in this relationship Dorothy were carrying all the anger and I all the "niceness." They confronted me repeatedly with my own hidden anger, which was squirting out in sneaky ways.

With their help and challenge, I took the risk of beginning to recognize and claim some of my own anger, which had been locked up for a long time. I took an even greater risk, or so it seemed to me at the time, in beginning to meet Dorothy's anger head-on with some forceful anger of my own. We had what I now look back on as some glorious shouting matches.

The results have been interesting and gratifying. Though Dorothy won't say that she likes my anger, she does like my being present to her. It is as if her energy no longer sails out into a vacuum, but is met by energy coming back from me. At that meeting place, a lot of life, love and fun are generated. I have also learned that sometimes her anger is a mask for pain, and that if I simply put my arms around her and hold her lovingly, she "melts" and leans into comforting from me.

This clearly has been a major theme in our life together, and an important theme in my development as a person and as a man. The successful work we have done in realigning our relationship has had important implications for my other relationships---to our children, my clients, students, colleagues and friends. It has made a great difference in my life, one that I am both grateful for and proud of.

As you will learn shortly, my inward journey has opened doors to even deeper dimensions of healing in our marriage.

Killing Cells

With Jean as my guide and accomplice, I made this imagery journey deep into my bone marrow. There I made the stunning discovery that these cancer cells were somehow *female*. This old issue, of the powerful, frightening female, I thought I had worked through and resolved. But here it was coming at me at the very cellular level of my body. These female figures, these bulbous cells, were out to do me in!

Later, people in Group 17 urged me to develop a warrior image to do battle against these dangerous cancer cells. I came up with a kind of Robin Hood figure, who held a special sword with a magic tip that could puncture and deflate a cell easily, and the sword's sharp edge could cut through the papery texture of these cells with no trouble. I bought and mounted on the wall of our bedroom a skeletal chart showing the areas of the bones where the myeloma was most likely to be active, and set about doing a kind of systematic sweep. In my mind's eye I would cut and slash my way through hundreds or thousands of these white cells, leaving their tattered remnants on the ground.

But it wasn't long before I began to have trouble with this imagery work, and the trouble was that I got tired. Even though this work was all in my imagination, the very notion of swinging that sword back and forth for hours on end brought on an imagined but very real fatigue. In addition to that, those cells had a discouraging propensity for reassembling and reforming behind me not long after I had swept an area clean. It was like trying to sweep out the ocean.

I was back in Jean's office, talking about my discouragement with staying at this kind of imagery work, when it suddenly dawned on me, and I said aloud to her: "I'm not using my best resource for this work. I'm not using my 'Brute.'"

"Brute"

Here I need to make another detour to introduce a long-lost part of myself who has come to be a key player in this narrative. Some ten years ago, after my first myeloma diagnosis but long before the second, I attended a workshop on visualization led by David J. Grove.[8] I volunteered for a demonstration with him and found myself sitting facing a large group of other therapists with David beside me asking some gentle non-intrusive questions about what I was now experiencing. I had been with David on a couple of other occasions, and had come both to trust him and to be much impressed with his artfulness in helping people elicit metaphors that illuminate their inner psychic process. I had no specific agenda in volunteering, but believed it would probably be interesting and valuable. Good prediction. Our exchange went like this:

David: "What are you aware of?"

Bob looks around, looks inward, checks his sensorium, and says: "I am aware of the cool air from the air vent up there blowing gently on my arms."

David: "And what is it like, having that cool air blowing gently on your arms?"

In the next three or four exchanges with David in which he essentially invites me to follow my awareness and describe it, I begin spontaneously to visualize a bare room with full-length open windows and long filmy white curtains blowing in the breeze.

David: "And what are you aware of now?"

Bob (long pause): "I'm aware of a kind of prickly feeling in my eyes."

David: "And where exactly in your eyes do you feel the prickly feeling?"

Bob: "In the back of my eyes."

David: "And what is that prickly feeling in the back of your eyes like?"

Bob: "It is like little needles."

David (now using one of his bridging questions): "And what might you be able to do with little needles?"

Bob: "I could get some thread and sew."

David: "And what might you sew?"

Bob: "I could sew a gown."

And I did. I took some of the filmy curtain material from the windows and sewed a gown which I draped over myself, and began to glide around the room. I became a beautiful woman in a graceful sweeping dance. In a little while I felt a pleasant fatigue, and imagined lying down on a pallet with the robe over me and going to sleep.

As I finished describing all of that to David and the group, he suggested that we now break for lunch, and come back to it in an hour. During the lunch hour I was in a kind of contented sleepy daze while I ate with a good friend. I didn't try to dissect this vision, as one might in analyzing a dream, nor have I really done so since. I have been content to let that vision be what it is, recognizing that the beautiful woman is an aspect of what Jungians would call an *anima* figure. I have met her two or three other times within me, and have come to cherish and value her place in my psychic life.

We reassembled after lunch, and David and I appeared again before the group. He didn't try to theorize about what had happened, or ask me to do so. He started again with a question about what I was now aware of. This time I had no clear awareness as I had had in the morning with cool air on my arms. This time I had only a hint of an elusive thought, and after a long pause I said:

"It's as if I could just barely catch a glimpse of something out of the corner of my eye."

David, going with the metaphor: "Which eye?"

Bob, surprised by the question, but instantly knowing the answer: "My right eye."

David: "And what might that be like that you can just catch a glimpse of out of the corner of your right eye?"

Bob: "It seems to be a box."

I went on to see and describe a box: about four feet on each dimension, made of rough boards, with only the front side visible in the light, and the back still hidden in the dark.

"I believe there is an opening or a door in the back, if I can get around there to see it."

Once more David interrupted the process, this time to suggest, given this illustration of how the evocation of a metaphor can work, that the group now divide up in pairs and practice the skill. I had no trouble picking up with my friend and partner, Roz, and with her skillful help was able to continue a puzzling and fascinating exploration.

I jockeyed the big box out into the light so I could see all around it, and found that it did not have an opening or door after all. It was nailed shut all around. And there was something inside it. In the spaces between the rough boards I could glimpse an ape-like creature of some kind--- dark, hairy, grunting, shuffling, sniffling, stinking.

I didn't know whether to be frightened or not. I didn't know whether he was frightened or not. I seemed to know that he was male---but that was all I knew about him. Did he want out? That would seem likely, but then I thought: maybe he has been *in* there so long he doesn't know what *out* would be like. Maybe *out* would be dangerous for him; maybe he'd wander across the street and be hit by a truck. I peered into the dark box, watching his small red eyes looking back at me, as if both of us were trying to solve a mystery.

After a time my partner, Roz, who had been listening to my puzzled description, made a suggestion, following another of David Grove's "bridging" strategies:

"Why don't you bring your other metaphor into contact with this one and see what happens?"

So I brought the graceful dancing woman from the other scene into this scene, and she glided gracefully back and forth in front of the box. Quickly I became uncomfortable with that event. For this beautiful woman to be swishing her ass around in front of this trapped primitive male creature seemed at best a bad idea, at worst cruel. It was like Fay Wray teasing a King Kong who was hardly bigger than she and who could not escape his bonds. Hardly fair.

So I sent the graceful dancing woman away, and again got down on my knees close to the box---peering in, trying to understand the mystery here. After a pause:

Roz asks: "What are you aware of?"

Bob: "I am aware of a prickling feeling in my eyes."

Roz: "Where in your eyes?"

Bob: "At the back of my eyes."

Roz: "And what is the prickling feeling like at the back of your eyes?"

Bob: "It is like there is an empty space behind my eyes, a sort of oval-shaped empty space with a gray mist in it."

Then with an awe-struck voice I said, "I am supposed to know about that creature in the box, and I don't know about him because there is a *hole in my head.* There is a hole where I am supposed to know about him and don't. And it is *not my fault.*" (That last sentence seemed very comforting to me.)

This was an awesome moment. I was in the presence of a powerful, mysterious creature who had something to do with me, and I didn't know about him till now. I also thought: my father was supposed to introduce me to this part of myself, but he didn't know how to do that because he didn't know this part of himself either.

That was enough for one day. As Roz's partner I helped her with some of her imagery, and then went home in a kind of daze. I had the creature with me, but I had no idea what to do with him.

Brute in Group 17

By happy chance, my Group 17 met a few days later. As I told them of my experience, they got excited and were quite certain about what they thought I should do with him:

"Get him out of the box," they insisted.

They were pushing me faster than was my cautious inclination. But I must have trusted them to protect me, or the creature, or themselves. Whoever most needed protection I wasn't sure. I got an imaginary crowbar and pried off the top boards and watched him climb out.

"What's his name?" somebody asked.

"Brute," I answered instantly, without any idea where the word came from. "His name is Brute."

Joseph, the group leader, invited me to escort Brute around the circle and introduce him to each of the members in turn. A strange and wondrous experience. "I want you to meet my Brute," I would say. I was holding Brute's hand, or paw; and I would slouch and rock and growl and make like an ape myself. It was wondrous fun, and deeply solemn and serious at the same time.

The most electric part of the experience was with the women in the group. Each responded similarly: as I would introduce Brute, her eyes would open wide (fear? excitement?), her face light up and glow with energy. Later most of them reported it was indeed a turn-on experience for them, for they had never before seen me so potently masculine.

By the time I had completed the circuit with fourteen introductions of this alien beast, he had become less alien, more at home in me and I with him. I took him in, and have relished him since as a valuable, long-lost part of myself.

About that same time, I came upon Robert Bly's story of *Iron John*,[9] about the hairy man at the bottom of the pond. I knew in an instant that Bly was telling my story.

Brute at Work

Back at my imagery work in Jean's office, I said to her, "I'm not using my best resource: I'm not using my 'Brute.'"

So I summoned Brute and turned him loose, in the theatre of my imagination, on these floods of cancer cells. What he was able to do was amazing. He sailed in and grabbed four or five of these big inflated figures in a great bear hug. He squeezed all the air out of them in a great "whoosh!" and they collapsed and slid to the ground. Then he grabbed some more and repeated the process. He seemed to love doing it---this is what he was made for--- and he carried on without fatigue and apparently without rest.

I didn't even have to monitor Brute. Whenever I would check in with him, there he was busy hugging and

squeezing and deflating bunches of cells, and more than
able to stay ahead of them, no matter how fast they were
reproducing.

When I felt like a little workout, I could pop down
there and join him by grabbing a couple of these big cells
and giving them a squeeze, listening as the air goes out,
and watching as they slid defunct to the ground. Brute and
I would grin at each other and have at it for a while; and
then I would bid him good hunting and take off to attend to
other matters.

I should mention that by this stage in my relation to
Brute, his appearance had changed a bit. His hairy pelt
had given way to more human skin, he was very muscular,
and his stance more upright. He looked more like, say,
Arnold Schwarzenegger. But like the original Brute, or
the early Arnold, he was still not much given to words.

Where Are the Healthy Cells?

After this important recalling of Brute, I was back
in Jean's office, telling of Brute's work in combatting the
cancer cells. I came upon another realization that I shared
with Jean in words like this:

"Knocking out these cancer cells is only half of the
job: I also need to be getting some action going with the
healthy white cells in order to beef up my immune system."

So Jean asked me: "Where in the scene of all this activity are the healthy white cells?" I looked around and fi-

nally saw them in the background---lying, as it were, against some kind of wall. They were behind the more active cancerous cells and easily escaped notice. These cells were smaller---about the size of a volley ball or soccer ball ---gray in color, and distressingly inert and inactive. They seemed to be just lying there doing nothing. And then another realization: these were *male* cells. Holy smoke! Another piece in this life drama---the passive, inert male.

So I talked to them to try to get them moving: "Come on guys. I really need you to get active."

Nothing happened. I felt helpless and frustrated at this point. How could I get these healthy cells moving, to be doing what I needed them to be doing?

Then Jean made a suggestion: "Why don't you go over and examine one of those cells more closely and see what you can find out about it?"

So I approached one of the cells, picked it up and held it in my hands. As I did so, it began to glow with a strange interior light, to luminesce like a pearl. My feeling changed from impatience to awe as I realized that something immensely precious was here, perhaps some kind of life inside this sphere waiting to come out. Maybe it was like an egg. So how could I help it hatch or come to life?

Jean suggested, reasonably enough, that I consult Brute. So I took the pearl/egg over and put it in his hands to see what he might make of it. Not much, and he passed it back to me with a kind of puzzled look. I said to Jean, "I think I need a female nurturing figure to bring this egg to life."

"Do you have one?" she asked.

After a moment's pause I said, "Oh yes, I do have."

Diana

What I was recalling then is an aspect of a Jungian *anima* figure I have encountered within myself on two or three notable occasions, one of them being the experience with David Grove in the workshop described earlier---a couple of hours before I found Brute. She appeared as a slender, graceful, shy young woman of beauty and poise, with a gentle curiosity and affection for the world around her. I now think that she was probably a part of my mother that got stifled and suppressed early in her life, in a manner similar to that in which Brute got buried in my father and in me. At any event, I have come, after a lot of initial nervousness and suspicion, to appreciate and honor and enjoy this feminine side of myself.

What I did then was to summon this figure. She showed up in a form I will name Diana---a kind of wood nymph with long golden hair and a simple flowing dress. I put this white cell sphere in her hands, and she did something with it that quite surprised and astonished me: she enfolded it in the fabric of her gown, and then pressed it into her body so that it somehow passed right into her lower belly. Then in a few moments she gave birth to a baby boy.

Diana then sat and held this child in her arms in a loving and tender way, and I was gazing at them both in wonder and awe. I became aware of a kind of golden light flowing down on this scene from above, and it occurred to me that this was like a nativity scene: Mary and the Christchild.

I was both inside this scene, like Joseph the father, and also outside it, observing it from a distance. I was suffused with a feeling of love and peace and joy. I reported all this to Jean as I was experiencing it, and left the session with a profound sense of awe.

By the next time I saw Jean, though, I had begun to ponder a puzzle: What is the relation between the emergence of new life from this one cell (pearl/egg) and all those other healthy white cells that needed to be animated? I had got one of them alive, but the others seemed still to be lying there, inert and motionless. Something else needed to happen here. What was it?

Jean and I pondered this together without much resolution. Then my life and work took another turn.

Achterberg and Lawlis

I came across an audio tape of a workshop presented by Jean Achterberg and Frank Lawlis, dealing with imagery and healing. This is an area in which the two of them have done a lot of interesting work.[10] I had met each of them briefly in the past when they lived and worked in Dallas, had read some of their books, and was now reminded that they might be the kind of resource I needed to help with the unfinished parts of my imagery work. I made bold to call Frank at their new home in California, was glad to learn that he remembered me, and told him that I wanted to get some consultation from him and Jean about my imagery. He said they didn't normally work with individuals that way, but suggested that I consider enrolling in one of the workshops they were planning to offer at Esalen that summer. I followed that lead by getting a catalog from Esalen, and enrolling in a weekend workshop on imagery and healing in late May.

Esalen is a whole story in itself: for more than twenty-five years a Mecca for growth-seekers of all stripes. It is a quiet retreat center on the beautiful rugged California coast at Big Sur, south of Monterey and Carmel. Along with other aspects of the human potential movement, Esalen went into some decline in the 1980's but is making an interesting comeback now. At any event, it had long been a wish of mine to visit Esalen, and this seemed like the right time.

About twenty people were in our group that weekend, and Frank and Jean introduced us to a number of interesting modes of facilitating healing through use of sound and movement and group ritual, and other aspects of what they generally describe as "shamanic resources."

I had an opportunity to share with the group something of my imagery work with my cancer, telling them much of what I have written here.

The group seemed much interested in what I was telling them, and asked me many questions about my experiences, including some of the same questions I was asking myself. How, for example, does this "nativity" scene relate to the energizing of the other healthy white cells? I said I didn't know and had come there looking for help with that.

At that point, Frank came and stood beside me and guided me into a couple of new experiences, the second of which turned out to be astonishing. First, he had me close my eyes and rock back and forth from one foot to the other. He stood beside me and rocked with me with one arm around me, the rocking having a rhythmic quality. He then invited me to imagine going into each of the two scenes, watching what happened.

The experience of rocking back and forth fit very nicely with the scene in which Brute was carrying out his campaign because it felt somewhat like marching in place, as in a military operation. Brute and I found that the rhythm worked very well in our crushing the white cancer cells.

But in the other scene the rocking seemed very much out of place. The mother and infant were very quiet, in gentle repose, and for me to be standing there rocking back and forth felt like a kind of agitation, a nervous twitch. So that didn't fit. I opened my eyes and reported this to Frank and to the group.

Frank then offered me something else. This time he had me place one hand on my stomach and the other on my upper chest, and he placed a hand on each of mine. He asked me to close my eyes and begin to hum. I started off humming on a fairly deep note, thinking, "Let's make this a manly hum." Each time I would take a breath and start a new hum, I raised the pitch a bit, and discovered that I could keep the tone going longer with a higher pitch. So over several breaths I raised the pitch, step by step. I could feel my energy rising as I was doing this. Later Frank reported that as he was humming along with me, he could at the beginning hold a breath through two of mine, but by the time I finished, he was breathing twice for each breath of mine.

What was happening in my mind's eye during this humming seemed to me quite wonderful. I saw myself standing by the mother and the baby, and singing to this newborn child. I was singing to him about what it means to be a man in this world. I don't know any of the verbal content of that song, but I was singing to him very precious information---all the things he would need to know to make his way in the world. This infant child could have been my own son, or he could have been my own infant self. Whoever he was, I was singing him into his being.

I am reminded, as I think of this, of Bruce Chatwin's writings about the Australian aborigines who sing enormously elaborate songs that are in effect aural maps of vast stretches of their territory, and who say that their forefathers "sang the world into being."[11]

So I was singing this newborn into his being. I said later to Frank that my father didn't sing to me. I think I didn't sing much to my sons and daughter. I am not yet clear how to describe what that means---for a father to sing or not to sing to his children. But it strikes me as a powerful metaphor for a precious form of fathering---to sing one's children a welcome into the world. Probably mothers do better with that---at least with lullabies.

As I was singing, I noticed something else happening. The energy of my song was flowing into these other cells that had been lying inert against that back wall. They began to glow and they began to buzz and they began to move---to lift, bounce, jump and fly about. Hosts of them began to fly this way and that. Some of them would go to where the empty husks of the old cancer cells were lying on the ground or floor and, like Pac-men, they would gobble them up. I had wondered previously how these empty husks were going to be disposed of, and then I found out. I could feel this buzzing energy flowing through my whole body, coming alive, vibrating with a wonderful zip.

So I came back to my home in Dallas feeling energized and alive in a new way. And I can recover that sense of alive energy pulsing through my body whenever I bring that scene to mind, whenever I revisualize that experience.

Achterberg and Lawlis II

In consultation with my wife Dorothy, I decided to go back to Esalen for the five-day workshop offered by Jean and Frank in August. This time I had a less clear agenda, since I felt I had accomplished my goal the first time in finding a way to round out my incomplete imagery work. But I was intrigued by other things that Frank and Jean were offering in their shamanic rituals. It seemed a good investment to have another round with them. What happened this time was less dramatic in terms of new insight, but very powerful as a new kind of communal experience for me.

About twenty people were in this workshop, only one of whom had been in the other with me. Frank invited me to tell the group about my cancer and about my imagery work, as I have reported it here. Again, this group appeared much interested in my account, and were quite ready to participate in a healing ritual that Frank and Jean set up for us.

I was asked to stand in the middle of the room with Frank close by my side; members of the group gathered around us. They were invited to touch or pat me in whatever ways seemed loving and appropriate for them, and to join me as I closed my eyes and started humming again. The humming filled the room with marvelous sound. We played with varying pitches and harmonies, and the volume and energy grew and grew. Then I found I could no longer contain the sound within me behind closed lips, so I opened my mouth and let the sound come out and soar to the ceiling.

I am still not sure how to describe the sound I heard, or if there is any single word to characterize it. It was high-pitched, with some of the quality of a scream, something like a wail, something like a yell of triumph, something like a battle cry. Other mouths opened and voices joined mine and rocked the room. I thought afterward that that first cry from me might have been like the anguished cry of a newborn infant, outraged at being thrust into a harsh world he hadn't asked for. But the cry flowed quickly into a kind of triumphant sound, a victory cry, a warrior's exultation. And as the group milled around me, joining in the cry, patting and touching me, sharing in a triumphal song, I began to feel like a newborn being welcomed into a sacred tribe. All these were my parents, my siblings, my grandparents, my cousins, my nephews and nieces, and many distant relatives---all united in kinship and love, giving thanks for my birth, welcoming me and singing me into my new life, and celebrating the birth and life.

So I returned from my second visit to Esalen with a richer and deeper gift. When I take myself back to that experience, I can both feel and hear within my body and spirit this pulsating song of life.

Couple Therapy

Toward the end of 1992, Dorothy asked if she could join me in the therapy sessions with Jean, and I was glad to welcome her into that process. She had been trying to deal with her fears and other feelings about my terminal illness, and had reported feeling very much an "outsider" with regard to my imagery journey. She wanted to be more than just a by-stander, and I was pleased about that.

Dorothy and I have been able to talk openly about the course of my illness and prospects for the future, and I have been immensely grateful to her for her courage about all this. She has not asked me to avoid or tiptoe around taboo topics like cancer and dying, and that freedom has been a great gift to me.

It was not a surprise to learn that Dorothy wanted to join in the therapy process. But it was a surprise to learn that my illness has stirred up for her some old issues from her past that were troubling but not easy to get at. These had to do with her shaky esteem as a female, and her need for affirmation and cherishing as an attractive and intelligent woman. This wasn't exactly news to either of us, but both of us were surprised by the flood of feelings that emerged with that awareness.

This is the big issue in Dorothy's psyche that corresponds to the big issue in mine, the struggle we have wrestled with over the years. We have done so well in growing and in healing wounds that we were surprised to

find how much of that pain is still in Dorothy, as I have
been surprised to find my issue dramatized in my cancer
imagery.

Jean commented on this process in two very helpful
ways. She drew my attention---kindly, but firmly and fre-
quently---to ways in which she saw me speaking and be-
having to Dorothy in unloving and inattentive ways, right
there in the office. That was unsettling because it confounded my belief that I had become the kind of husband
Dorothy needed and I wanted to be.

But I couldn't refute the examples Jean would point
out to me, often minor but telling: how I would look away
instead of toward Dorothy, miss the pain in her words, josh
her about something tender---events of that order.

Each confrontation startled and dismayed me.

"Why am I doing that?" I asked.

Jean responded, "Why are you doing that?"

She then gave me an assignment for the week:　I
was to get a pad of paper, find a quiet place and quiet time
to sit down and write about this question.　In the assignment, I was to bring that question into the context of my
journey of discovery so far.　Had I learned anything there
that might help me with it?

I don't know all that Jean had in mind in making
that assignment, but it led to a remarkable discovery.　As I
began to think and write about Dorothy and about my imagery work, it dawned on me that in spite of all the good
work that she and I had done in healing our relationship, I

had still been imaging her in my mind as the powerful female I had to wrestle with. I had done well with that, as described earlier in this narrative, and a lot of energy, fun, eros, and love had been generated in that wrestling. I had come from a long way back in overcoming my timidity and passivity, my knee-jerk tendency to retreat or placate. I have described here some of how I learned to overcome that, to locate my inner anger and force, and to meet Dorothy with it face-to-face when appropriate.

(That is what I think Robert Bly means when he speaks of "Zeus energy." My finding my inner Brute has helped me claim my "Zeus energy.")

Hera and Diana

In Jean's assignment, as I reflected and wrote on these matters, it came to me that I was continuing to image to myself Dorothy in the form of this powerful formidable female. Perhaps I could call her Hera, in Greek mythology the wife of Zeus.

I will come back to Hera in a moment. But to follow my reflections, I need to report that at the very moment I saw myself imaging Dorothy in that way, I also saw that I didn't have to: I could picture her in a different way. I could see her as Diana.

It is difficult to describe the jolt of wonder and awe that accompanied that emergent picture. In my mind's eye I could see Dorothy as Diana---the graceful, tender, gentle, beautiful woman, cherishing and loving her son into his manhood. There is nothing false about that picture---all those are qualities that Dorothy has in abundance. What shifted for me was that I brought that picture forward on the stage of my mind, and let the picture of Dorothy as Hera recede to the background.

As I did that, a major internal shift occurred: I felt my heart open toward Dorothy in a new way. In following days, I found myself thinking about her lovingly at odd moments. I realized that in truth I was safe with her. I had come to believe that with my head, but apparently never before with my heart.

As long as I was picturing Dorothy as Hera in my unconscious mind, it made sense never to quite relax my guard. Zeus and Hera, in the Olympic legends, were a great and glorious couple, possessing great and passionate devotion, but also fiercely competitive and capable of god-awful (I think that is the precise word I want) rages and battles. Love---but be on guard.

I awoke to the discovery that I did not have to hold the Hera image. I could choose to visualize Dorothy as Diana. A remnant of something hard and resistant melted around my heart in that moment.

For two weeks I kept this discovery to myself---playing with it, watching Dorothy, watching myself, floating with this new inner sense. At our next session with Jean, I thanked her for the assignment and reported what I had found. And I told Dorothy for the first time about now seeing her as the Princess Diana, and something of what it meant to me.

Dorothy was startled, cautious, even troubled by my disclosure. She had considerable difficulty taking it in.

She asked, "Does this mean I have a new image I am supposed to live up to?"

"No," I answered, "it doesn't mean that you have to do anything. You have just become Diana for me in my way of looking at you."

Dorothy's acceptance of this new view of her was slow coming, occupying several counseling sessions. She said one day: "I have been longing all my life for you to be in love with me. Now that it has happened, I am so over-whelmed I hardly know what to do with it."

In months that have followed, two aspects of this phenomenon have impressed themselves upon me as re-markable. The first I might call the power of the image. Dorothy becomes different when I image her as different. My heart opens to her in a new way when I see her in a new way.

This idea will not be strange to "constructivist" so-cial theorists or to quantum physicists, both of whom are at home with the idea that we "construct" the realities around us---even in certain ways the physical realities---by the way we see them.[12]

The second fascinating thing I noticed was how much more Diana-like Dorothy has in fact become---

touched and softened, as it were, in the warmth of my new way of relating to her.

Changes Diana-ward have occurred at both levels: in my new picture of her, and in her new way of being in response to that. Hard to separate those.

We both feel blessed and grateful, and are aware that this journey of discovery was stimulated by the death sentence of multiple myeloma. I doubt I'd have made much of the journey reported here without that ominous summons. Shall we offer thanks for the cancer? That may take more grace or courage than either of us can muster right now. But without question, we are both immensely grateful for the new gifts it has brought.

The Dance

Now to the most important passage in my imagery journey---the discovery of the dance. It happened in response to a suggestion from another friend and professional colleague, Donald Weaver. After reading an earlier draft of this manuscript, Don said to me:

> "You have two archetypal female figures in your imagery work, Hera and Diana, and you also have two male figures. The first is 'Brute' who is powerful and knows well what he is doing in containing and squashing the cancer cells. The other male figure is not as clear as 'Brute.' He starts off as a newborn nurtured into his life by Diana and sung into his manhood by you. He transmits the energy of his life into other healthy white cells, but he hasn't himself taken much form as a

grown-up male. Wonder what he will look
like and act like as an adult male?"

With that intriguing invitation, I made some quiet
time and re-entered the stage of my inner drama. There I
watched, and was enchanted by something I had no conscious preparation for. This young man, fully grown, full
of masculine grace and energy and force, came to the
scene where Brute was busy squashing the cancer cells.
What the young man did was to take one of these cells in
his arms and begin to dance with it. He whirled it around
in a graceful spin. As he did that, an amazing transformation began to occur in this great bulbous balloon. It
changed shape---shrinking its bulk, articulating arms and
hands, legs and feet, hair and face of a beautiful woman.
Now there were more couples like this, dancing, swirling
around the floor, which became like a great Viennese ball-
room---Strauss waltzes surging through the air, the space
awash with whirling, swirling couples---a fantastic ongoing wonder of movement and music and energy.

The embarrassing truth is that in real life I am a
most clumsy dancer. But in the theater of my imaginary
bone marrow, I am Fred Astaire and Rudolf Nuryev. And in
this scene I have multiplied beyond number. I have become a multitude, dancing with my cancer cells and
changing them into beautiful women.

In former months, when I would check into my
bone marrow, I would find Brute busy there, squashing
cells right and left, and sometimes I would join him for an

invigorating workout. I know now that was an important and necessary stage in the development of this imagery drama. But it was not an ending place.

This dance scene may not be an ending place either, but it feels much like the right healing place. In Brute's scene there is mostly silence: only the whoosh of escaping air from the cells and the occasional satisfied grunt from Brute.

In contrast, the dancing scene is sensorily very rich. The eye is enchanted with swirling color and movement. The ear is awash in floods of music. And the body pulses with the joyous rhythm of the dance.

So now when I "check in," I am swept up in the dancing. The dance with cancer becomes what looks and sounds and feels like the dance of life itself.

To repeat what I have said, or at least implied before, about these imagery scenes: I don't have to *make them happen*. I didn't consciously invent them, nor do I have to *crank them up* to re-enter them. And now, of course, the richest scene is the Viennese ballroom where the dance of transformation is going on all the time somewhere inside me. I think it important for me to look and listen in on that scene, to feel the surge of that marvelous energy in my body, every day for at least a few seconds or minutes.

An elegant reminder of that pleasant assignment was given me by Dorothy in the form of a tape of Strauss waltzes. I play some part of that each day as I drive to and from work, and delight in my mind's eye with the glorious pageantry of the dance.

TWO

REFLECTIONS

"Life can only be understood
backwards, but must be lived
forwards."
--Soren Kierkegaard

Survival

What can a reader expect to make of this narrative so far? What do I make of it?

Both questions interest me very much, and I am far from certain of the answers to them.

Certainly I hope that this story may be of use to readers who struggle with serious illness---either as patients or as helpers concerned with patients. My story obviously can't be a blue-print or a road map for another's journey---it is too unique, too personal, to serve that way. But my hope is that it can be an encouragement and stimulus to a reader to explore some of his own pathways to self-discovery and self-healing.

As for my own assessment of this story: Do I believe that my imagery work has significantly affected the medical course of my cancer? Yes, I do believe that. In the next chapter I will show laboratory data to support that belief. But belief, however plausibly supported, is short of proof in a scientific sense. So I want to be careful to distinguish those, and not make fanciful claims.

We need to start with the fact that multiple myeloma runs a quite variable course in different patients. About half of all patients do not respond to treatment and typically die within a year or two after diagnosis. Other patients respond well to treatment and survive for varying periods. *Wintrobe*[1], a well-known textbook on hematology, reports a median survival time of between two and four years from the onset of therapy. Another source says that a ten-year survival period is remarkable. Another reports twenty years as the longest known survival period.

At this writing, late 1994, I am nearly fifteen years past first diagnosis and completing nearly four years of active chemotherapy. At this point, I am still symptom-free, and my blood scores continue to improve. (See chapter *Three*.)

My oncologist, Robert Burns, is pleased with these results, and likes what I have shared with him about my inner journey. He has a hard time believing that any kind of mental activity can have much direct effect on cancer activity once it gets under way. But he believes that whatever leads to inner harmony and sense of well-being supports healing in general. So he encourages me in this project, but cautions me not to get my hopes too high.

Mind/Body Mystery

My doctor's advice is reasonable enough. We both know that we are working here in a place of great mystery: the overlapping area in which the realms of body and spirit interact. Lots of attention is coming to bear on these matters. Witness Bill Moyers' recent book and video series on *Mind and Medicine*,[2] the popularity of books by Bernie Seigel, Depak Chopra, Larry Dossey---all medical doctors, by the way---and a host of other material too rich even to catalog, let alone to summarize here.

What is possible to say about this mysterious mind/body relationship is that there are two positions clearly and obviously wrong:

The first derives from the classic Cartesian split between mind and body. In this view, which essentially underlies Western scientific medicine, the body is a complicated machine running by its own rules. It is affected by intruders like germs and viruses, and by internal malfunctions and break-downs, but not significantly by attitudes, emotions or intentions of the person-in-the-body.

That view gets tougher for all but the most hidebound medical technicians to hold to. Floods of information about such matters as the placebo effect, newer research on psychoneuroimmunology, added to anecdotal accounts from all ages of medicine, tell us that the Cartesian boundary is very porous indeed. It leaks copiously in both directions.

But there is an equally absurd position that oversimplifies the complex mind-body relationship in the opposite direction. This view in effect dissolves the Cartesian boundary by holding that the body is a kind of extension of the mind without its own autonomy. Christian Science is an institutionalized form of this nonsense (peace to my Christian Science friends), and it shows up currently in a number of "New Age" cosmologies. In such views, one wills one's illness, though perhaps unconsciously, and thus can will it away. If I change my attitude, image the right images, pray the right prayers, meditate the right meditations, I can make the deadliest disease go away.

If I don't succeed in doing that, it means I didn't do it right. So I get to bear the double curse: of making myself ill, and then failing to make myself well.

Both these extreme positions seem to me preposterous. Somewhere in between is the great fascinating area of mystery and possibility.

What Heals?

I believe this imagery work has been effective in combatting and healing my cancer. In the next chapter I will present some data that support that belief. But before presenting that material I want to assert that this work, whatever its outcome medically, has been healing and life-giving for me as a person.

I live with a kind of dilemma here. The "outcome" of my work---prolonged health and well-being, absence of symptoms, and so on---I do take as confirmation of the validity and importance of my self-healing work. "Daniel Boone" has discovered new territory.

On the other hand, I am reluctant to tie the work and the medical outcome too closely together. I believe the work has come to have its own power and validity, no matter what the course of the cancer. It has changed my life

in profound ways. I like to think that this imagery journey can stand---or shall I say "dance"---on its own feet.

I know that in the beginning the imagery work was
important because it gave me something to *do*. I remember well that famous article, later a book, by Norman
Cousins, called *Anatomy of an Illness* [3] about his life-
threatening collagen disease. He found a number of important things to do, including laughing at Marx Brothers
movies, to get himself actively into cooperation with his
doctor's medical treatment.

To feel helpless, totally dependent on the power of
another to preserve or protect one's life, is a place most
people find scary and demoralizing. Maybe there are ex-
ceptions. Maybe there are some for whom that can be a
neutral or even comforting experience, relief at turning
the keeping of one's life over wholly to another.

When I had my heart by-pass surgery five years
ago, I was by necessity in that kind of helpless place for a
while, and I believe I managed it with some grace. In the
recovery room after the surgery, I could do little for myself. I even had a tube down my throat to breathe for me.
It wasn't easy, but I was able to accept my essential helplessness and dependency on the competence and goodwill
of the people assigned to my care.

My point is that while life may on occasion deal us a
hand like that, I don't welcome it. And I don't have to see
my cancer that way, a game in which the doctor has some

cards to play but I have none. I am going to look for and play whatever cards I can find.

To follow the metaphor of "game" and "cards," just what kind of "game" is this? What is this cancer about?

Disease as Teacher

I was startled to discover in my visualization work that the cancer cells appeared to be threatening female forms. It is as if I were being confronted again at the microcellular level in my body with an issue that had been a major issue in my life pilgrimage.

Why now? I had thought I had that worked out. Was there some part of it not finished, that still needed dealing with?

The more recent developments in my imagery work suggest that the answer is "Yes." I have been led to explore my relationship to Dorothy more deeply, and to make important changes there. New dimensions of living in the real relationship have in turn opened up new aspects of the imagery work. I seem to be moving back and forth in a synergistic way between healing in my body and healing in my relationship, each supporting the other.

So I could answer: Yes, it does seem that there is a lesson here for me to learn, one that I wasn't aware of, or thought I had finished with, until the cancer scared me into looking for it.

But if there is a valuable lesson for me to learn, must we then ask who or what sends the lesson? On that question my jury is still out. None of the conventional answers to it make sense to me. I don't see God sending the cancer, for either punitive or pedagogical reasons. Nor does it seem useful or sensible to me to say that I brought this cancer on myself.

What I can safely say is that I have been presented in a new way with a picture of a major drama in my life, and have been challenged to tackle it with as much vigor, courage and imagination as I can muster. I have been like Daniel Boone, striking out---or better, striking inward--- to unknown territory. What I have found are surprising things I didn't anticipate, including perhaps some real healing of my "incurable" cancer, and certainly including a new loving partnership with Dorothy.

Disease as Metaphor

A larger question can be asked at this point. Suppose we grant that there seems to be here a significant parallel between the "form" of my disease and the "form" of my life. Is there anything we can generalize about that? Anything applicable to someone else's cancer or someone else's life? For example, do other myeloma patients have life issues like mine with the powerful female? I would be fascinated, but also quite surprised, to find that to be true.

Until recently I had met only one other myeloma patient, a middle-aged conservative Protestant minister. When I shared with him an earlier version of this manuscript, and asked if there were a powerful female issue somewhere in his life, his response was astringent. He reported that as a youngster he had a mother somewhat threatening and overpowering. But it was important for him to let me know that in his adult life he has been no wimp. His congregation and his family recognize him as a strong leader, a take-charge guy, who doesn't let others run over him---certainly not women. Testimony noted.

"Killing" Cancer

My journey has prompted me to think long thoughts about the nature of cancer itself, and the way we talk about it. Our discourse about cancer, both public and private, tends to bristle with military and battlefield metaphors. We talk about "fighting" cancer. For more than twenty years we have been in a government-funded "War Against Cancer." Ironically, except for notable small victories, the overall story is that we are losing the war. Carl and Stephanie Simonton, who first brought imagery work to public attention in cancer treatment, often encouraged their patients to image a kind of inner battle scene, with the radiation or chemotherapy as good soldiers or warriors destroying the bad cancer cells.[4]

That, by the way, is not an inaccurate metaphor for much cancer treatment. In my case, the chemotherapy is a kind of killer. It is a poison (cytoxan, one of those agents derived from mustard gas) that attacks all the cells in my body. Cells are most vulnerable when they are dividing, and cancer cells divide more quickly than healthy cells. Thus the right dosage of poison knocks off lots of cancer cells, with tolerable---and reparable---damage to healthy cells. In those terms it certainly sounds like a war: keep killing them before they kill you.

But even from the beginning I have found that warfare imagery is an awkward fit with the idea of cancer. One of the things we can say about cancer is that it is a form of the *life process gone awry.* In the development of any organism, cell systems are coded to know when to divide and reproduce themselves, and when to stop dividing and reproducing. If a system doesn't reproduce enough, it will show up as a developmental deficiency, as in birth defects like cleft palate or spina bifida. If the system doesn't know how or when to stop reproducing, then the unlimited growth becomes itself destructive of the integrity of the larger system. Cancer tumors are clusters of cells that didn't stop growing when they should have. They have forgotten how to die. If my disease progresses, the out-of-control proliferating cancerous white cells in my bone marrow will in time crowd out the healthy white cells and red cells. The end of that process will be destruction and death. But it is interesting that that process begins with the life force itself---the impulse to growth. These cancer cells are a part of me that once worked to protect me. They were a part of my immune system, attacking and devouring alien invaders. Now they have lost direction and control and are banging around inside me, have themselves become "alien." Surely in ideal terms, the goal of cancer therapy would be to find some way to bring this powerful, out-of-control life force back into harmony with the whole.

Out-of-Control Systems

That idea may not be as far-fetched as I first assumed. In the next chapter I will report some findings about new directions in cancer research that seem to point very much in that direction. But in this section I will follow my intuition about healthy and unhealthy systems, and speak of things I have learned in psychotherapy and family therapy.

It is not uncommon to encounter a family in which a youngster has gotten "out of control." Imagine a four-year-old, with parents who for reasons of ignorance, insecurity or indifference have never learned to say "no" to him. Such a child will almost certainly become a tyrant, rendering everyone's life a misery, including his own. In this social system, this child is a form of the life force gone out of control, dominating the family and inwardly terrified of his power to do that. The treatment goal with such a family in therapy would be to help the parents take charge and establish appropriate limits and controls. Then the youngster may be able to climb down from the exhilarating and terrifying position of being in charge of everyone, and can then find his more healthy and structured place in the family

I find the analogy intriguing, and it fits with my own imagery journey. As that journey finally comes to the scene of the glorious dance, with cancer cells being re-formed back into life-giving forms, a true integration is achieved.

My discomfort with battle-field imagery, and my fascination with the image of the dance, draw me to consider another analogy from the realm of psychotherapy. Would-be clients often show up in the therapist's office with request for help to get rid of something they dislike about themselves. I have been that route myself. What I have learned is that therapy seldom works that way. The surgical metaphor, "cutting something out," may be useful in some areas, as in blocking an addiction. But for the most part, therapy which aims at excising some part of the personality turns out to be frustrating and ineffective. What one tries to "get rid of" usually sticks like Velcro. The opposite is also true: what one tries to hold on to, like happiness, is likely to slip out of one's grasp.

Genuine therapy is about opening up and adding things, expanding choices, not about contracting, subtracting or amputating things. It usually proceeds by one having the courage, or grace, to own and embrace the rejected part---the "shadow," in Jung's terms.

"To embrace the rejected part." That phrase has deep resonances in Biblical and other religious traditions. It is what showed up in my own internal imagery work, where Brute's assault on the cancer cells is replaced by a dance in which those deadly cells are transformed.

Dancing With Cancer

Dancing itself is a multi-layered and fascinating metaphor. The image of the Dancer came to me *sui generis*, of itself, without conscious derivation from anywhere else. But as I contemplate dance, thoughts about it crowd my mind.

Dance can be seen as a metaphor for the most fertile and creative relationship between male and female. Dance both requires and creates energy in the interplay between the two partners. Think of Fred Astaire and Ginger Rogers in any of their movies, or Al Pacino and his partner tangoing in the movie "Scent of a Woman."

By convention, which may have roots in evolutionary biology, the male usually takes the initiative, inviting the female into the dance. If she accepts the invitation, her part then becomes a subtle and fascinating blend, or alternation, of resistance and compliance. If there is no resistance, there is no spark or energy in the dance. She becomes simply a passive figure moved around by her partner. Remember the comic gyrations of Donald O'Connor with the life-sized rag doll, reprised in the movie "That's Entertainment"? It was very funny, but not really a dance---only a burlesque of one.

For the dance to be really alive requires the ever present possibility of the female dancer's resistance, either by leaving or pushing back. If she leaves, the dance is over, at least for now. If she pushes back too strenuously, the dance stops flowing and becomes a fight. If her resistance, either in trying to leave or push back, is overwhelmed by the male's counterforce, then it ceases to be a dance and becomes something else---a violation or rape of some kind.

For the dance to be aesthetically and kinesthetically satisfying, it has to embody some dynamic interplay of those opposing vectors: resistance and compliance, conflict and confluence, pushing against and flowing with, fighting and yielding, Hera and Diana.

Dances, of course, vary in the way they balance these vectors, and the degree to which they make that polar tension overt and explicit, as in the Apache dance, or just implicit, as in graceful ballroom dancing. But I suggest that the dynamic is present in all vital forms of male-female dancing, and similarly in the most interesting and energized forms of male/female relationships.

Back to my bone marrow: appearing here is the surprising image of dancing with deadly cancer. These destructive agents of the life force gone awry are restored to their "original" form. They are partners in the dance of life.

THREE

BLOOD LEVELS

Cancer Levels

If one has to choose a cancer, multiple myeloma offers at least one major advantage: as a blood cancer, it is easy to monitor. Its advance or retreat can be measured easily by routine blood tests as often as desired. On the charts following I have gathered and tabulated information about the course of my disease and our treatment of it. The findings are interesting and encouraging.

As I have reported before, myeloma can run a quite variable course. About half of all patients do not respond to treatment and typically die within a year or two of diagnosis. Those that do respond to treatment live an average of two to four years. My prolonged good health, as shown in the following charts, is not wholly without precedent, but puts me for now in a very small class of unusual survivors.

Chart 1 shows two indices of cancer activity: Immunoglobulin G levels, measured in thousands, and SPE Protein levels, measured in integers. Since the myeloma cancer cells remain in the bone marrow, they are not measurable directly. But these proteins produced by the cancer cells do circulate in the blood where they can be counted. They provide an indirect but reasonably accurate measure of the cancer activity. In this chart both lines show a significant decline.

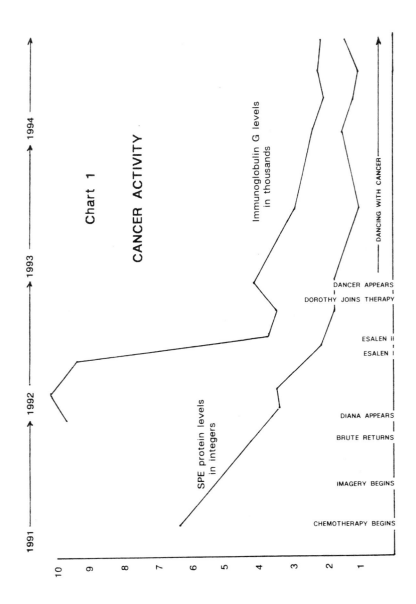

Chart 1

CANCER ACTIVITY

1991 1992 1993 1994

SPE protein levels
in integers

Immunoglobulin G levels
in thousands

DANCING WITH CANCER

DANCER APPEARS
DOROTHY JOINS THERAPY

ESALEN II
ESALEN I

DIANA APPEARS

BRUTE RETURNS

IMAGERY BEGINS

CHEMOTHERAPY BEGINS

10 9 8 7 6 5 4 3 2 1

The most striking thing about Chart 1 is the precipitous drop in IgG levels at mid-1992. That corresponds to the time between the first and second visits with Jeanne and Frank at Esalen. Is it possible that what I did with Frank in that first visit could have had such an impact on my cancer? That was when I first got into the humming and imagined myself singing this newborn child (my infant self? my infant son?) into his life and manhood. That was an emotionally powerful experience. Could it have kicked the cancer back like that?

The Believer in me says, "Sure, why not?"

The cautious Skeptic in me says, "Wait a minute! I'll tell you why not: because the imagery and the scale don't match. The imagery work with Frank was not about kicking cancer, but about birthing and nurturing the healthy white cells, keeping my immune system up and running."

"Well," says Believer, "then let's turn to what we can see about the white cells."

That brings us to Chart 2.

White Cell Levels

Chart 2 is a good deal more dense because it includes two notations for almost every month over nearly four years. Unfortunately it doesn't speak very directly to the question about my work with Frank, but it does suggest that the Dancer is a potent force.

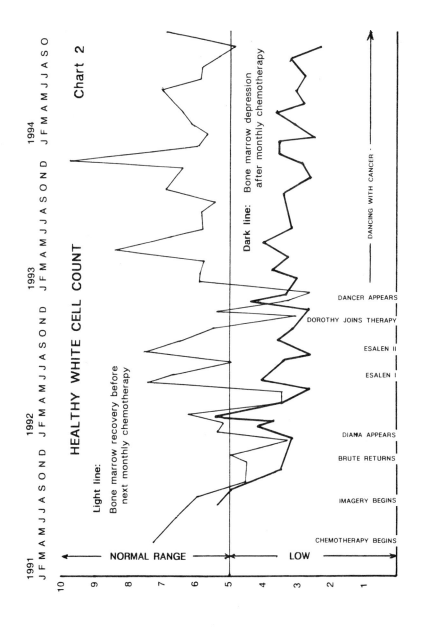

Chart 2

HEALTHY WHITE CELL COUNT

Light line: Bone marrow recovery before next monthly chemotherapy

Dark line: Bone marrow depression after monthly chemotherapy

The scores on the left of the chart are in thousands. Above the line at 4.8 is considered normal; scores below that line show immunological risk. My doctor measures those levels twice a month and watches them carefully; they tell him how hard he can safely hit me with the chemotherapy. He wants to kill cancer cells with the stiffest dose that won't take out too many healthy cells.

My doctor reads this blood count before and after each monthly five-day round of chemotherapy: thirteen days after completion and then just before the next round. Thirteen days after is considered the danger point, when the white count is likely to be lowest. On the chart these are the dots connected by the heavy line---almost all below the "normal" line. By the beginning of the next five-day round, it is hoped the system will have recovered to a safe level of white cells. These scores show on the chart as dots connected by the light line, mostly above the "normal" line.

Thus, it is a good sign when the dark line hovers in the low range, because that means the chemotherapy is *working:* it is killing cells. It is also a good sign when the light line hovers up in the "normal" range, because that indicates that in each of these months there is a restoration of healthy white cell activity. Some lively restorative process appears to be at work in my body.

Two places on the chart show such a positive effect. The first is in 1992, from May to September. This includes the time of my work with Frank at Esalen. But I have to confess that I don't find the chart easy to read here. The scores before and after that period are so scattered as to be confusing. So I will let that go by and invite the reader's attention to a less confusing place on the chart: 1993 and 1994.

Restoring White Cells

From January 1993 onward there appears to be a consistent, clear and significant recovery every month. All the post-chemotherapy (heavy line) scores are in the 2's and 3's, low enough to be in the danger zone. But each of those scores is followed by another (light line) score well up in the normal range. It would certainly seem that something has been active in my body restoring my damaged immune system for a long time. Could that something be the Dancer(s)?

Believer says, "Sure, that feels right. That is exactly the time when the Dancer has been active."

Skeptic says, "Wouldn't that be interesting if it turned out to be true; and how would we know for sure?" Skeptic goes on to say, "Although these figures seem to bring the imagery work and the doctor's work closer together, there is still not a very precise fit."

Consider: the Dancers transform cancer cells back into healthy (and beautiful) white cells. What a happy solution! But is it reasonable to think that something like that literally happens in the physiology of the blood? Isn't it more plausible to think that the ratio of healthy to malignant cells is changing because more good cells are produced and more bad cells are knocked back? In that case "transformation" would remain a loose metaphor rather than a literal description.

Biological Response Modifiers

I was content to live with that loose metaphor mentioned above until the summer of 1994 when a startling conversation opened up with my oncologist, Dr. Burns. We were looking at my blood scores, which have continued to be impressively healthy.

Dr. Burns asked me, "Do you think the Dancer is doing that?"

I said, "Sure. Have you got a better explanation?"

He answered, "No, but I just don't have a theoretical frame that I can put that in."

A generous statement from a no-nonsense doctor. My cautious inner Skeptic can appreciate his difficulty.

Then I asked him another question: about this loose metaphor, the Dancer, changing cancer cells to healthy cells.

"I presume that that does not correspond to what actually happens in the blood," I said. "It must be that cancer cells die out and are replaced by healthy ones."

"Don't be too sure about that," he said. "Your metaphor may be more accurate than you realize."

He went on to tell me, with some enthusiasm, about what he sees as the oncology of the future in the development of what are called biological response modifiers.

"Our major current treatments for cancer are barbarous, if you stop and think about it," he continued. "We attack the body with a knife in surgery; we burn it with radiation; and we poison it with chemotherapy. If artfully done, and if the body has enough recuperative resources, sometimes the cancer can be checked or destroyed, and the patient recovers from this assault. But it remains a barbarous assault.

"The hope for an oncology of the future---and it is now beginning to appear---lies with agents we can call biological response modifiers. These have the capacity to attach to the surface of cancer cells, penetrate the cells, and alter the internal chemical/physiological process of those cells so that they cease being malignant.

"This research is still in its infancy. The two best known such agents are Interferon and Interleuken-2. They can have heavy side-effects, and are effective only with certain cancers. But they point to a future oncology that will be very different from what we have now."

So here is an unexpected confirmation that my Dancer image, who changes ugly cancer cells to beautiful women, may not be as fanciful as it would seem.

It certainly is exciting to me to think that my unconscious mind may be stimulating my body in some mysterious way to produce its own biological response modifiers.

In the meantime, my oncologist and I are continuing with the "slash and burn." I take chemotherapy every month, a medication that "kills" healthy cells as well as cancer cells. Isn't there a sharp contradiction between the idea of killing cells and the idea of transforming them?

Of course there is, but for now I am going to live with that contradiction in trust that some resolution may appear.

Ruthless Immune System

Perhaps the immune system itself can offer a clue to what such a resolution of the above-mentioned conflict might look like. The immune system embraces a similar paradox: in order to heal, it has to kill. Its job is to keep us alive, and without it we'd all be promptly dead, knocked off by the first bad microbe to wander into our body. It protects, preserves and enhances life. What a lovely upbeat, constructive piece of work that is.

But take a second look. The immune system goes about that task with a ruthlessness that, viewed on a human scale, would be shocking. An alien germ crossing the border is met, not with a polite request for his passport, or temporary internment while his status is reviewed in court, or even deported back whence he came. No, he's dispatched with a shot between the eyes! Or, in what's a more accurate (and grosser) image, he is eaten alive---cannibalized. Those white cells just gobble him up.

So my immune system is a precious friend who uses bloody tactics to protect me. Even if I knew how, I would not want to teach him to be non-violent.

If that paradox of killing and healing is there at the very cellular basis of life itself, maybe it is not crazy to believe that the goal of transforming cancer into health may include bloody and violent tactics like chemotherapy. Perhaps that is not an elegant solution, but it is a clue worth pondering.

FOUR

Where's Brute Now?

"I see the balance of my life---everything comes in images now---as a beautiful paisley shawl thrown over a grand piano.

"Why a paisley shawl, precisely? Why a grand piano? I have no idea. That's the way the situation presents itself to me. I have to take my imagery along with my medicine."

--Anatole Broyard[1]

Out of Work

Here is a brief story that rounds out my narrative journey. I could have added it at the end of chapter *One*, where that story culminates in the glory of the dance. But I think it deserves a space of its own. It is connected to that journey, but its emergence in the theatre of my mind came only after a long interval---almost eighteen months.

It is about Brute. What has happened to him?

When the Dancer(s) appeared, Brute's work was superseded. It was taken over and transformed into another mode, the wonder of the dance. For a long time I had been so enchanted by the vision of the dance that I had in effect forgotten Brute or ignored him. Well, not quite. Every once in a while a whisper of conscience would remind me of my debt to him and suggest that I go look for him. But the prompting was not urgent and I put it off.

Until recently, when my old friend, John Schaffer, got after me. John is a pastoral counselor in St. Louis who has developed an interesting model of guided imagery[2] in his practice. I had opportunity to spend a day with him after he had read a form of this manuscript, and he pressed me about Brute

"Where is he? What has happened to him? Have you abandoned him?"

I had to admit that I didn't know Brute's whereabouts, but agreed it was time to find out. So with John's help I went looking for him: relaxing, closing my eyes, journeying inward on the quest.

It didn't take long. I found Brute in the back of the Viennese ballroom in a kind of hallway, leaning against the wall near an exit sign, looking quite disconsolate. I asked how he was doing, and he answered, "I don't have any place here. My work is done. It's time for me to leave."

I felt alarmed. I didn't know where leaving would take him, but I urgently wanted him to stay. But what could I tell him?

I finally got his agreement to hold steady for a bit. I went over to and interrupted one of the dancing couples. I told the young man that Brute might be leaving, and he came over to Brute with an even more urgent plea: "Please don't go. You don't seem to know how important you are in this place. *If it weren't for you, we couldn't do what we are now doing in the dance!*"

The young dancer didn't have a clear explanation of exactly how that was true; but I could hear the conviction in his voice, and I believed him.

"If it weren't for you, we couldn't do what we are doing. You ought to have a place of great honor in this room."

Brute heard these words and thanked him for them, but seemed quite unconvinced. He continued to look sad and lonely. I didn't know what to do. I had to let him be where he was and struggle with what he was struggling with. I left the scene, telling him that I wanted to come back and talk with him again.

Two weeks later, I met for lunch another therapist friend, Tom Simpson, with whom I have shared parts of this story. I told him I had reached a stuck place with Brute, and was hoping that he, Tom, could help me find a way through that.

As Tom listened, I began to set the scene, describing what I have set forth here. Before Tom had a chance to open his mouth, I had a startling new vision, and burst out:
"He is the *Godfather*!" I told Tom.

The Godfather

Piece by piece, as the scene unfolded, I told Tom what I was seeing. Brute now looks like Marlon Brando playing Don Corleone in his declining years. He has still the residue of enormous controlled force in his shoulders and trunk and in his sagging jowls. In his eye can be seen the occasional flash of menace. But he has softened and mellowed. He looks out on this gorgeous room full of dancers. These are his sons and their wives, his daughters and their husbands, and children and grandchildren. And he knows he made all this possible. They can dance because he was once ruthless enough and strong enough to kill---when he saw it as necessary.

It is not necessary now. He takes a few turns in a clumsy, funny parody of a dance, and then retreats with a smile. The dance is just not his game. But it is the game he made possible. The dancers smile and bow to him as they pass. In his chair of honor, he smiles at them, and nods. And dozes.

****

The Evolution of Brute

This evolutionary development of Brute I find fascinating and awesome. He began, if you will remember, a primitive hairy ape-man whom I found nailed up in a rough box. With the help of Group 17 I got him out and began to befriend him, to own him as a part of myself.

Some seven or eight years later I called on him to help me fight the cancer cells, and he proved a whiz at that. By that time he had lost his fur pelt, stood upright, and looked and sounded more human.

Now at the finale he has become the honored Godfather, progenitor of the dancers, looking out on them with pride, enjoying the scene of wonder and beauty he has made possible.

Where, in the mystery of my unconscious, did all that come from? My interest in Jung invites thinking of that as an archetypal journey, grounded in something more deeply and universally human than just my own private personal pilgrimage.

Maybe in time I will come to believe I know more of what it all means. I have a hunch that Robert Bly could tell me some interesting things about this story; maybe some of my readers can too. I'll leave it there for now.

FIVE

Thoughts About Life and Death

"The wonder, and the terror, and the
exhaltation of being at the edge of being."

--Anatole Broyard [1]

Contrary Truths

A paradox lies at the heart of this book. A paradox consists of contrary truths that somehow have to be held together. The contrary truths to be held together here are that it both is, and is not, important that I survive a long time in my "dancing with cancer."

It is important for me to survive because that validates my story, makes it "true," demonstrates that imagery can be effective against cancer. Unless I can really show that, what's the point of telling this story? Part of me certainly believes that, has much invested in expectation of long life, of thereby winning the battle.

On the other hand, another part of me knows that longevity is beside the point, that the story either validates itself or not. It is not about long life; it is about dancing. Dancing doesn't have winners and losers. It is not judged by how long it goes on, but by what happens in the dance. This journey of discovery has transformed my life and my marriage. If I were to die before this story sees print, the story is still worth telling.

So it both is and is not important that I survive a long time.

This is not the only paradox I have found myself pondering in recent months. Dr. Johnson's dictum about a sentence of execution intensely concentrating the mind

has certainly been true for me. It has energized my attention in two directions:

(1) coping with this deadly disease, and

(2) pondering what is important about life.

These two can intersect, as in the renewed awareness that
only in the here and now can life be truly lived. The only
space and time we have is here and now, and each day can
be welcomed as itself a miracle. I find that realization
challenging, consoling, healing.

Coping

I have searched for literature on how others have
coped with cancer and found a lot of it. There is little on
multiple myeloma itself, but many anecdotal accounts describe "conquering" or "overcoming" or "defeating"
deadly cancers by varieties of "alternative" treatments,
often after orthodox medical treatments were judged to
have failed.

I have found these narratives helpful in varying
degrees. Least convincing were the "here's-how-to-do-it"
narratives: "Here is what I did to conquer my cancer: if
you follow these ten steps, you too can be healed."
However healing occurs, I think it is likely to be more
complex and mysterious than any ten steps.

Saying that reminds me of my inner qualms about
publishing this story. I have been urged by friendly readers to believe that telling this story can be helpful to oth-

ers, and I want to believe that that is true. But can it be of help?

I certainly want to believe that my story can be an encouragement or a guide to others. But it is obvious that this is a long way from a "how to" book. There is no simple way for me to teach another to follow the kind of path that I have been on. I didn't even teach myself in a conscious way. I opened myself to being led. With the help of Jean and other wise coaches, I allowed myself to be guided by a source of inner wisdom deeper than I consciously knew. I don't have a clear name for the source of that wisdom. Wearing my Jungian hat, I could call it the wisdom of the Unconscious. Wearing my Christian hat, I could call it the Holy Spirit. Wearing my Eastern hat, I could call it the Tao. But how could I teach someone else to access that Source?

I want to believe that I can. Some of my psychotherapy clients have been able to use guided imagery and visualization to profound effect in unusual ways. Now that I am beginning to work with some cancer patients, I am feeling more hopeful about my ability to be such a helpful guide.

Spontaneous Remissions

Some patients with serious diseases die sooner than they "should," gauged by their medical condition. Other people live longer than their medical condition would predict. Some even recover completely from deadly cancers for reasons that baffle their doctors. When reported, these cases are called "spontaneous remissions."

Recently Brendan O'Regan of the Institute for Noetic Sciences tracked down medical references to some 1500 such reports and was able to find full case reports of some 430 of these.[2]

O'Regan wanted to bring this mysterious and fugitive material into the light where it could be studied, to see what might be learned from it. He readily acknowledges that the task is formidable: most of the reports are tantalizingly brief, limited to medical data alone, and usually bare of information about the personhood of the patient. Even from as many reports as he found, it is hard to draw useful generalization

Other physicians like Bernie Siegal[3] and Larry Dossey[4] report interesting stories of unusual cancer recoveries. Many of these accounts describe the importance of what might be called "spirit," a certain kind of buoyant attitude toward the disease and toward life. This attitude would seem to include courage, determination, hopefulness.

But even these qualities can appear in quite different form. Larry Dossey tells of one of his patients who treated her cancer diagnosis as a kind of rude interruption of more important matters, such as tending her roses. With tremendous concentration of will she attended to the richness of her busy life, and treated the cancer as an impertinent annoyance, beneath notice. As if properly chastised, the cancer did seem mysteriously to slink away for many more years than would have been expected.

At the other end of the coping continuum are stories of people who bring their lives to a screeching halt at the time of diagnosis. They turn in radically new directions: change jobs, leave spouses, throw over old life styles and adopt new ones. Many of these stories have positive outcomes.

Maybe even courage comes in different forms. For some it is courage to stay the course. For others it is the courage to change the course.

Courage, spirit, determination to fight do seem to characterize survivors. But there is a contrasting quality that also appears in many of these accounts---a quiet sense of tranquility or peace, a calmness in the face of deadly threat. This is not resignation or despair, but a kind of affirming acceptance of what is. These survivors seem to have found what Deepak Chopra means when he says: "Complete healing depends on your ability to stop struggling."[5]

Polarity

Survivors would seem to need to struggle and to stop struggling---another kind of paradox. The mystery of healing would seem to involve a strange polarity, a balance of opposites: fighting against and flowing with, resisting and accepting, attacking and embracing. Such a polarity seems very close to the metaphor of dancing I found in my own imagery journey. The dance is a conjunction of two contesting energies, each having the potential to wound the other; but together they create a new energy of beauty, power and harmony.

The most thoughtful presentation of polarity in healing I have found is in Ken Wilber's *Grace and Grit*.[6] This book is an elegant, eloquent and moving account of his five-year marriage to Treya, which ended with her death from cancer. Her first diagnosis came two days before the wedding; so fear, sadness and joy were mixed into their marriage from the very beginning. Between them they already knew a great deal about the extraordinary resources of the human spirit. Wilber has written a number of highly regarded books bridging psychology and spirituality and Western and Eastern philosophies.[7]

Ken and Treya tracked down and tried a number of "alternative" cancer therapies as well as conventional radiation and chemotherapies. I opened this book with some dread because the book jacket told me the ending was not a happy one. But once into it, I could not put it down. It is the wisest and richest book about living and dying with cancer that I have found.

The title, *Grace and Grit*, itself suggests that polarity of fighting against and flowing with. An even richer phrase is one coined by Treya, "passionate equanimity." She writes:

"I was thinking about the Carmelites' emphasis on passion and the Buddhists' parallel emphasis on equanimity. This somehow seemed more important to me than the age-old argument about theism versus nontheism that these two groups usually engage in, and which seems beside the point to me. It suddenly occurred to me that our normal understanding of what passion means is loaded with the idea of clinging, of wanting something or someone, of fearing losing them, of possessiveness. What if you had passion without all that stuff, passion without attachment, passion clean and pure? What would that be like, what would that mean? I thought of those moments in meditation when I've felt my heart open, a painfully wonderful sensation, a passionate feeling but without clinging to any content or person or thing. And the two words suddenly coupled in my mind and made a whole. Passionate equanimity, passionate equanimity---to be fully passionate about all aspects of life, about one's relationship with spirit, to care to the depths of one's being but with no trace of clinging or holding, that's what the phrase has come to mean to me. It feels full, rounded, complete and challenging." [8]

Passionate Equanimity

I love that phrase, passionate equanimity, and am grateful to Treya for it. I aspire to live my life by it.

I want to live life passionately, to cherish and embrace life with an ongoing sense of excitement and wonder.

And I want also to be able to "sit loose" to life, to observe it in all its absurd complexity with a kind of benign, detached, amused curiosity. And I want to be able, when the time comes, to let it go without regret or fuss. One of my favorite mantras is this: Everything is interesting and nothing is important.

I like to play golf with passionate equanimity. When I am waggling my three-wood at the ball and eyeing the green 190 yards down the fairway, every molecule of my body is invested passionately in the planned trajectory of that ball. Nothing else in the universe matters. Then, if the ball curves off into the bunker, I like to be able to say with equanimity something like: "Well, that's interesting. That will test your skill coming out of there, Bob."

Passion and equanimity. If not quite simultaneous, at least in rapid alternation.

My oncologist and I seem to be winning right now in this battle (hard to escape that word, even when I don't like it) against the myeloma, and I readily own being excited and grateful for that. On the other hand, when I am thinking clearly I know that the victory is temporary, and that all in all it's not terribly important how long I live. "Healing" is about "making whole," and the wholeness of life includes its ending in death. It both is, and is not---as I said at the beginning of this chapter---urgently important that I survive. Granted, that's easier to say now at seventy-three than it would have been at thirty-five or fifty, or even sixty.

I remember waking in the middle of a troubled sleep a couple of years ago, and hearing a voice from somewhere deep inside me say: "I am not willing to make death the enemy, or dying a defeat." I heaved a big sigh of relief and went back to sleep.

I don't want to sound naive or sentimental about dying. Sherwin Nuland in *How We Die* [9] suggests that it is seldom peaceful or easy. Information about multiple myeloma suggests that the end of that process is likely to be painful and grim. I may do a lot of wailing. But I like to think that I will be ready to relinquish life gracefully and gratefully when the time comes.

The Fear of Life

Auntie Mame said, "Life is a feast and most poor sons-of-bitches are starving to death."

I believe that much of the fear of death is really the fear of life. Because life comes packaged with pains and dangers of various kinds, people often try to hold it at arm's length. Then when the game is over and the bell rings, they may panic, as the life they haven't let themselves live slips away and they try desperately to cling to it.

It's hard to give up what you haven't let yourself have. It is hard to let go of what you have not loved.

Like Treya, I aspire to love life passionately, to work for it as long as I am able, and when the candle flickers, to relinquish it gratefully.

APPENDIX A

Complementary Treatments

for Cancer

"It is much more important to know
what sort of a patient has a disease than
what sort of disease a patient has."
--Sir William Osler

Office of Alternative Medicine

In 1992 the National Institutes of Health, under some prodding from the U. S. Congress, established an Office of Alternative Medicine.[1] Its director is Joe Jacobs, a physician with interesting credentials for leading the National Institutes of Health into such "uncharted terrain." He is by birth a Mohawk Indian, with medical degrees from Yale and Dartmouth, an MBA in health care administration from the University of Pennsylvania, a commission in the Public Health Services, and practice experience in the Indian Medical Center in Gallup, New Mexico, where two worlds of medicine meet everyday. In 1993 the Office announced some thirty research grants, totalling nearly a million dollars, for study of non-conventional forms of medical treatment, including some for cancer. The list of grants embraces a remarkable range: guided imagery and hypnosis for cancer, acupuncture for attention deficit disorder and unipolar depression, macrobiotic diet for cancer, even prayer intervention for substance abuse. [2]

Though these grants are a minuscule fraction of the budget of the National Institutes of Health, the very existence of this office is a signal emblem of a new climate in the health care field.

Climate of Discourse

Following my first diagnosis of myeloma back in 1980, I searched out as much information as I could find about treatment options for cancer. It wasn't easy to sort through. What I found were mostly polarized and polemical broadsides. A number of alternative "healers" and their supporters had formed advocacy groups, ready to accuse establishment medicine of selfish turf protection and callous disregard of patient welfare. Official medicine often returned the compliment by describing unorthodox "healers" as unscrupulous fast-buck artists preying on frightened and gullible patients. An anxious patient trying to find an objective and balanced overview had his work cut out for him.

As my initial scare about cancer receded, I eventually turned attention elsewhere. Eleven years later, in 1991, after another diagnostic wake-up call, I began to explore the literature again. I am glad to be able to report that, at least in some venues, the quality of discourse has considerably improved. Though one can still find plenty of vituperation and calumny (I love those words!), one can also find serious and responsible attempts to build bridges, to assess various and conflicting claims, and to offer readers some balanced information about what's out there.

The most valuable of all the sources I have found, by far, is a new book by Michael Lerner.[3] He is the president of the Commonwealth Foundation, a research and treatment center featured in Bill Moyers' TV series "Healing and the Mind."[4] Neither a physician nor a "healer," Lerner is a social scientist who has gathered an immense amount of information about various cancer treatments and treatment claims; he lays this information out in an objective and balanced way. The title is *Choices in Healing: Integrating the Best of Conventional and Complementary Approaches to Cancer.*[3]

Note the term "complementary." It has considerable advantage over the more familiar term "alternative," a term which suggests that one has to choose between this treatment and that. Once in a while such a split may be called for. But for the most part patients trying out other methods---like imagery, diet, acupuncture, meditation, and the like---are not abandoning their medical treatment but adding to it. Broader use of "complementary" in place of "alternative" would, I think, lift the quality of our discourse even more. Older usage hangs on, however. Even Lerner, who likes "complementary" and puts it in the title of his book, falls back in his text to the frequent use of "alternative." And Joe Jacobs' office researches "alternative" methods.

It is long past time for serious consideration of a multi-dimensional approach to cancer. For one thing, the official medical "War on Cancer," launched more than twenty years ago, has proved a misfire. Some marginal cancers have yielded to cure, but rates for the major cancers are advancing, not retreating. And the embarrassing news to medicine is that patients in droves are consulting other "healers."

In 1992 the *New England Journal of Medicine* published an article, "Physicians and Healers---Unwitting Partners in Health Care," by a physician and psychologist[5] arguing that patients would be better served if that unacknowledged partnership between physicians and healers were brought out more into the open and some attempt made jointly to establish standards for responsible treatment across the board. The authors cite a report by the Office of Technical Assessment, published in 1990, of a three-year study commissioned by a committee of the U. S. House of Representatives. The study found that one of every three Americans consults non-conventional therapies for illness: chiropractors, acupuncturists, psychotherapists, hypnotists, nutritionists, massage therapists, meditation teachers, yoga instructors and others of such ilk. Patients usually do not abandon their medical doctor or his/her treatment. But in many instances they don't tell their doctor what they are doing, for fear of disapproval. Another interesting finding is that such patients are not typically the poor and uneducated, as the medical myth would have it, but rather are more educated and better informed about their illness than the average patient. Most of these patients see what they are doing as "complementing" their medical treatment, not replacing it. That certainly has been true for me.

Psychological   Factors

I want to turn now to the area of complementary cancer treatments that could be called psychological or psychosocial. I have been astonished to discover how extensive and rich this literature is, though I must promptly add that the findings are often mixed or contradictory. A friend, Elias Baron, has shared with me his doctoral research paper entitled "Psychosocial Factors in the Etiology and Clinical Progression of Cancer: A Literature Review,"[6] in which he has cited over 125 sources. These are all solid research reports from medical, psychological or other responsible professional journals, beginning in the 1950's and accelerating into the 1990's. This field is getting increasing attention, with results that show many interesting leads, though the findings are still often mixed.

As Baron's title indicates, two general questions have been asked about the relation of psychology to cancer. The first is about etiology, or causation: are there psychological or emotional traits or experiences that predispose people to get cancer?   Put more dramatically, is there such a thing as a cancer-prone personality?

The other question is about the role of psychological interventions in the treatment of cancer. That question falls into two parts: (a) can such interventions reduce anxiety, raise morale, and otherwise improve the "quality of life" of cancer patients? and (b) can such interventions actually combat cancer and help patients get well, or at least survive longer?

Causation

I will address these questions in sequence, starting with the one about etiology. Here lies a fascinating history, going back as far as the birth of modern medicine with the Greeks. Galen, in the second century, wrote that breast cancer occurred more often in "melancholic women."[7] In the nineteenth century, many physicians made similar observations about cancer patients. The medical literature of that period has been reviewed and summarized in a fascinating way by the psychologist Lawrence LeShan in his book *Cancer As a Turning Point.*[8] He found that:

"... up to 1900 the relationship between cancer and psychological factors had been commonly accepted in medical circles . . ."

"I went through the major cancer textbooks of the nineteenth century (using the old rule of thumb that if it went through three editions, it qualifies as a major textbook). All but one of the nineteen I found said the same thing: 'Of course, the emotional life history (they used a lot of different phrases for this, but the meaning was the same) plays a major role in the tendency of the person to get cancer and in the progress of the cancer.'"[9]

These sources listed such factors as "great emotional loss, hopelessness, mental misery, melancholic temper, grief," and similar forms of "mental disquietude,"[10] as predisposing factors in the development of cancer.

By the end of the century this point of view began to fade from textbooks and journals and soon vanished completely, for which change LeShan offers two major reasons. First: surgery, then radiation, later chemotherapy, appeared on the scene to offer more effective medical treatment for cancer than anything heretofore available. The second reason LeShan proposes is the reverse side of that treatment coin. For all their plausibility, these psychosomatic views of the origin of cancer were hard to put to use. Nobody found an effective way to apply these insights to prevent cancer or to treat it once it arrived. This is a point worth pondering, and I will return to it later in discussion of more recent research.

By the 1950's new stirrings of interest in psychological approaches to cancer appeared, some of it attributable to LeShan's own psychotherapeutic work with cancer patients.[11] The theme has been taken up by others, even poets.

W. H. Auden wrote about cancer:

> "Childless women get it
> And men when they retire---
> It's as though they needed some outlet
> For their foiled creative fire."[12]

When Woody Allen in the movie "Manhattan" says, in effect, "In our family we don't get angry; we get tumors instead," we know that such an idea has again become current in the folklore of our time. Or perhaps it only went underground after the 19th century.

This idea had become current enough that in 1977 Susan Sontag published a brilliant and blistering critique called *Illness as Metaphor*.[13] Her major device is to compare the psychologizing of cancer in the mid-twentieth century to the way in which tuberculosis was viewed in the nineteenth. Readers of Dumas' *Camille* and Mann's *The Magic Mountain*, and viewers of movies about nineteenth century romances will recognize how often that disease was romanticised, and treated as a metaphor for certain fragilities of spirit or quirks of character. When antibiotics came in and brought tuberculosis under effective control, all that metaphoric discourse simply vanished. Sontag believes that that will also happen with cancer when effective medical cures for it are discovered. In the meantime, she argues, patients already frightened and demoralized by a diagnosis of cancer are subjected to the doubly cruel burden of being asked to believe that they brought their deadly disease on themselves by some defect of character or of personality.

That is a matter deserving careful and sensitive attention. I believe that any hypothesis about psychological predisposition to cancer needs to be separated into two questions: (1) is it true? and (2) if true, is it useful? My quick answer to the first question is: probably yes; to the second, probably no.

Is It True?

To start with the first question: More sophisticated and dependable measuring instruments have been devised than were available to nineteenth century physicians, who had to depend only on clinical impressions. Some of the more current findings are certainly interesting.

Starting in 1946, Dr. Caroline Bedell Thomas of Johns Hopkins University began following a group of thirteen hundred medical students, using psychological tests and personal interviews. In 1978, she reviewed her data and found that two hundred of the students had developed serious diseases, forty-eight of them cancer. The striking finding about the cancer patients was that they had mostly reported being not close to their parents in childhood, and had generally negative feelings about early family life.[14]

The science writer, Henry Dreher, has gathered data from a great many studies of this kind, and has summarized them in a chapter titled "The Psychological Factor" in his book *Your Defense Against Cancer*. He suggests:

> "People who go on to contract cancer often recall a difficult childhood, characterized by a lack of closeness to one or both parents. As a result, they feel alienated and alone, and often experience later difficulties in establishing close and fulfilling relationships.
> "Many cancer patients suffer a profound feeling of hopelessness and despair about achieving any meaning in life---whether from relationships, creativity, or work achievements. The feeling seems to have

existed long before any cancer was diagnosed. Often, it is present as far back as the patient can remember.

"The expressions of emotions---especially anger are characteristically suppressed or repressed. Such people....seem to deny their own needs and hold in their anger from an early age for fear of rejection by others."[15]

Type "C" Personality

The London psychiatrist, Steven Greer, in studying women with breast lumps, identified a construct he called the "Type C" personality. What principally distinguished women with benign tumors from those with malignancies was the frequency in the latter of "suppression of anger." They ranked lower in general on emotional expressiveness, but the statistical significance of the suppression of anger was greater than any other factor. In summary he wrote:

"A cancer personality picture beginning to emerge: People who are loathe to express disruptive or hostile emotions; people who tended to be 'awfully nice,' compliant and afraid to assert themselves."[16]

Lydia Temoshok, a psychologist at the University of California at San Francisco, has also developed data supporting the Type C hypothesis. She contrasts it to the Type A personality, which is at risk for heart disease. Type A's are chronically angry, Type C's chronically "sweet" and "nice." She and Henry Dreher have recently published

The Type C Connection: the Mind-Body Link to Cancer and Your Health,[17] in which they survey an immense amount of research around this issue.

In summary, I would say that it is hard to dismiss out of hand the weight of so many of these findings, though I have touched on only a few. In fairness it must also be said that many careful researchers have come up with results that fail to support the Type C hypothesis or similar ones. What seems reasonable is that with this hypothesis we are looking at a risk factor of some weight but not compelling weight. As Dreher says:

> ". . . probably more so for younger or middle-aged patients, than for older patients, in whom age-related factors---including the break-down of immunity that comes with age---seem more significant and psychological variables less so."[18]

Is It Useful?

Now to the second question: Even if there is some truth to the idea of a psychological factor in the etiology of cancer, is it a useful truth? Does it help patients, either before or after they get cancer? Here I am much more skeptical, more in sympathy with Susan Sontag's view.

Take my own case. In some ways, as chapter *One* makes clear, I fit the profile of the "nice guy," who spent a lot of energy in early life suppressing, or repressing, anger, discounting my own needs and deferring to the wishes of others. But it is also true that I have worked hard over the years at coming out of that corner. I have been known to refer to myself as a "reformed" (or in the current jargon, "recovering") "nice guy." But my motive in working out of that corner has not been to avoid cancer but to wake up and become more fully alive. It is hard for me to believe that any warnings about the danger of cancer would have had much effect on the course of that psychological journey.

In general I think fear, shame and guilt are poor motivators for change. They may serve as a wake-up call, an alarm-bell in the night: "Wake up! Something is not right!" But working at change requires something like hope and a vision of a new possibility. If someone with a Type C personality, who has learned to cope with stress by covering helpless/hopeless feelings behind a stoic "nice guy" or "sweet girl" front, is presented with a diagnosis of cancer, then I think he or she is more likely than not to respond to that jolt in precisely that way. Under stress we are more likely than otherwise to fall back on our familiar coping strategies.

Can "cancer-prone" personalities, once cancer occurs, learn to change their basic coping strategies in ways that can help them? That is a more pertinent and useful question to which I will now turn.

But before I leave this section, I want to note something about the Temoshok/Dreyer book that truly puzzles me. The paper edition is sprinkled on the front and back covers with testimonials from such worthies as Bernie

Siegel, Jon Kabot-Zinn, Dean Ornish and others on how helpful they think this book will be to cancer patients. Perhaps they are more careful readers than I. But what I read, while often fascinating as information, offered very little useful guidance to me as a patient. It is hard for me to imagine how other patients will find it useful.

Help in Coping

I turn now to the more useful question: can psychological resources assist cancer patients in coping better with their illness. Lots of data here suggest that the answer is clearly "yes." In the broad arena of mind/body medicine, still echoing with vituperative polemics, this seems to be the part of the arena least argumentative. Most cancer clinics or hospital divisions of any size provide "support groups" for patients, giving them a chance to ventilate feelings, gather information, share with fellow patients. Not every patient needs or wants such an experience, but many patients do and testify to the value of such groups.

Few physicians would discourage their patients from enlisting in such support groups, which are known to improve "quality of life" for many patients. But if a claim is offered that such groups can have a "curative" effect---can "combat" cancer or extend the life of patients--- the discussion suddenly gets testy again.

What seems to worry physicians about such claims are two fears: one, that patients will build "false hopes" that later collapse and leave them demoralized, or; two, that believing that you can assist in your own healing implies that you must have helped bring the illness on in the first place. There is a certain logic in both views, but I think both use false logic.

The first mistake---about false hopes---confuses hope with expectation. Hope means openness to (healing or redemptive) possibilities in the future. Read that way, no hope is *false,* because the future *is* always open to new possibilities.

Expectation, on the other hand, is an attachment to a specific content of hope. It may be, if not false, at least unrealistic in its investment in a specific outcome. More seriously, it may by such focus close off openness to other possibilities.

By defining too narrowly, for example, the kind of healing one "hopes" for, one may miss the gift of a broader and deeper kind of healing.

The second worry of doctors is that inviting patients to take some responsibility for their own healing implies that they must also thus be responsible for their own sickening. I am sure that there are patients who put it together that way, but the logic is faulty. If your house is on fire and you pitch in vigorously to help the firemen try to put it out, that does not constitute evidence that you started the fire in the first place.

Research on Group Support

A notable shift in this debate occurred in a 1989 report to the American Psychiatric Association by David Spiegel of Stanford University Medical School. Ten years earlier he and associates had studied eighty-six women with metastatic breast cancer, randomizing them into two groups. Both groups received the best available medical treatment. In addition, patients in the experimental group were provided opportunity for several months to participate in a weekly support group where they could talk to one another about their experiences and their feelings. Spiegel predicted, and found, that patients in these groups, as compared with the controls, coped better with their illness, had less fear, less pain, improved "quality of life." What he did not predict, and was surprised to find, was that the women in these groups lived longer. In follow-up studies ten years later, he learned that these women had lived an average of twice as long as the control patients.

These findings confounded Spiegel's own expectations, for he said he undertook the research partly to refute belief in the curative effect of such interventions with cancer patients. This skeptical stance, plus Spiegel's impeccable credentials in medicine, have given his findings an unprecedented weight in the cancer world. Michael Lerner calls it "a watershed event."[19]

Spiegel and others are now busy replicating these studies, and trying to sort out and measure the various components of that "support group" experience. Is it the talking that heals? The listening? Ventilating feelings? Developing friendship and care for others? Sense of sharing a common fate? Some or all of these in some combination? It is obvious that sorting out the variables is not going to be a quick or easy task.

It is interesting to note that in 1993 a report very similar to Spiegel's appeared from the medical school at UCLA. There Dr. Fawzy I. Fawzy and colleagues had some years before provided a form of group psychotherapy for a group of melanoma patients, matched with controls who got the same medical treatment but not the psychotherapy.

I quote Lerner about this report:

> "Fawzy's intervention was strikingly minimal. It consisted of only six structured 1 1/2 hour group sessions over a six-week period. The group meetings offered (1) education on melanoma and basic nutritional advice, (2) stress management techniques, (3) enhancement of coping skills, and (4) psychological support from the staff and from other group members."[20]

Six years later, at follow-up, Fawzy found, also to his surprise, significantly increased longevity and longer disease-free intervals for his subjects, compared to controls. It seems clear that psychosocial interventions of this kind show intriguing promise in the treatment of cancer, and ought to be investigated vigorously.

I myself am not surprised by these group support findings. In my own experience I have found group care and group support a powerful resource in my own life and healing. I have described two notable group experiences in my earlier narrative. One was with Frank Lawlis and Jean Achterberg at Esalen where my new "family" joined in singing me an exuberant "welcome into the world." My heart still leaps when I remember that. The other experience was the moment in Group 17 when I plummeted to the bottom of my feeling of helplessness. I have been thinking a great deal more about that event since reading a profoundly moving account of the life and death of another myeloma patient.

Andrew Greer

Such accounts are not easy to find, and I stumbled on this one by accident in the bookstore. It is titled *In Mysterious Ways: The Death and Life of a Parish Priest*, and was written by a journalist, Paul Wilkes. [21] The story is of an altogether exemplary priest named Andrew Greer. With affection and admiration, Wilkes for some years followed the work of Father Greer in the Boston area, where Greer won the devotion and loyalty of parishioners, peers and superiors. He is described as devout, bright, courageous, loving, gentle, firm---all the qualities of an admirable pastor and leader.

In 1987 came the ominous diagnosis of multiple myeloma. He faced that with courage and grace and managed the chemotherapy well for about three years until its efficacy began to fade. His doctors offered a more radical experimental treatment in the form of bone marrow transplant. After much deliberation, they decided to go for it. The transplant process, which I won't try to describe here, can be a harrowing ordeal, and it certainly was so for Father Greer.

The poignant and heart-breaking part of the story is not about the pain and anguish he endured, but about what happened to his spirit during that ordeal. The radiation knocked everything out of him, physically and emotionally---his health, his courage, his faith, his hope. When he was squashed flat, this dear man, who could reach out to hold and comfort other sufferers so well, had no way to open up to let someone else hold and comfort him. His faith was tied to an image of self able bravely to endure all things. When things became truly unendurable for him, he had no refuge. When friends came to solace him, he would either try to be brave or turn his face to the wall. He did leave the hospital and resume his ministry, but he had little heart for it. His image of himself had broken. He apparently believed that he had failed his God, his people, his faith, himself.

Father Greer lived for another two years, and, remarkably enough, his myeloma returned only in moderate degree. What he died of, in the opinion of at least one of his doctors, was depression.

I find this story profoundly moving and sad. It renews my gratitude for the way in which Group 17 was there to hold me when I needed them. When I had the courage, as it were, to let go of my *show* of courage, and to fall into that pit of fear, they went down in there with me, and I let them hold me. I am more and more reminded of what an important turning point that has been for me in my journey.

I trust I do not need to deny any intent to be critical of the Catholic priesthood. It may be true that the culture of training for celibate priesthood does not easily conduce to the experience of leaning on another for emotional support. But this is a matter more human than ecclesiological. I know Catholic priests who are able to own their own fragile humanity when up against it, and I know Protestant clergy and other helping professionals, married or otherwise, who are not.

Individual Psychotherapy

Individual psychotherapy has failed to chalk up much of a record of success in the treatment of alcoholism and other addictions. It has had to acknowledge, when honest, that AA and other 12-step programs are the treatment of choice.

The psychotherapy of cancer patients, with one exception to which I will refer shortly, seems to be about as much of a blank slate. Psychotherapists---like pastors, nurses, and other caregivers---can give important support and palliative care. But almost nobody has been able to develop and publish a testable psychotherapeutic model for helping cancer patients fight their disease.

The one exception I have been able to locate is Lawrence LeShan, a psychologist in New York (see reference to his historical research on page 95) who has been at this game since the 1950's. He has written ten books, including two on the psychological treatment of cancer, *You Can Fight For Your Life* and *Cancer as a Turning Point*.[22] Recently he has summarized his cancer work in a lively taped lecture.[23]

LeShan's story is of special interest to psychotherapists. What he brought to his initial work with cancer patients was the Freudian heritage he shared with most self-respecting therapists of the time. The Freudian model, LeShan says, invites the therapist to explore three questions:

(1) What is the presenting problem (symptom)?

(2) What is the hidden cause behind the problem?

(3) How do we resolve that hidden cause?

With lots of troubled people that model of psychotherapy is very useful. With cancer patients it is not, says LeShan.

It took LeShan a while to learn this, and slowly to evolve another therapeutic approach. The goal of his new approach is to enhance the immune system---the body's natural host-resistance to cancer, or any other disease. In this model the most useful question is something like, "If you were living out your (hidden) dream, feeling fulfilled, waking up in the morning excited to be alive, going to sleep at night happily tired, what would you be doing, what would be going on?" LeShan helps patients find or recall their (lost, unfulfilled) dream, find how to translate it into something possible, and then how to implement the plan.

The results he reports are fascinating. When he first began working with cancer patients in the hospitals, the only patients the doctors would allow him to talk to were those already considered terminal. In the first few years, using his Freudian tools, all his patients died. As he developed his new approach, some patients began to live longer. In time, he says, half of his "terminal" patients went into indefinite remission. He has fascinating stories to tell about patients' recalling and finding ways to live out their dreams---"learning to sing their song" is one of his favorite metaphors.

In some of the therapy work I am just now beginning to find my way into with cancer patients, I am realizing that LeShan's model is promising and exciting. And in interesting ways, I find it to mesh very nicely with the strategy of visualization, which has been the major dimension of my own healing work

APPENDIX B

VISUALIZATION

"I seem to have an awful lot of people inside me."

--Dame Edith Evans

Esoteric or Common?

Visualization for change, or guided imagery, has become more widely accepted and used in recent years. But it still may strike some readers as a strange phenomenon. Or it may appear to others as an esoteric technique available only to an adept few. For a reader in either camp, some further description may be help.

For openers one can point out some everyday experiences of visualization we all have.

If you should be asked how many windows are in the front of your house, chances are you will come up with an answer in the way most respondents do: calling up a mental image of your house and counting the windows. This is visualization.

Worry is a very common human experience depending on imagery. In order to worry, we have to visualize some unwelcome event in the future. In a corresponding way, guilt is about the past where we visualize---re-live in the theatre of our mind---some regrettable transaction.

But can mental pictures make changes in our body? Consider: when we chew food, glands in our mouth are stimulated to secrete saliva which assists mastication and begins digestion through an alkaline bath. However, a hungry person can usually start salivating just by imagining that he has tasty food in his mouth. How does that happen? How does the mind stimulate the salivary glands to produce? I doubt that we really know, though we certainly take it for granted that it happens.

Looking at a nude *Playboy* pin-up, or even just imagining that he is looking at one, can produce another kind of physiological alteration in a healthy male.

Now to more unusual examples: certain Indian yogis, after years of discipline and training, appear able at will to bring about marked changes in heart rate, blood pressure, blood flow, and other "autonomous" body functions. Many ordinary people, after a few minutes connected to a bio-feedback machine, will be able to produce similar results, though they usually won't be able to tell how they did it.

A subject in a hypnotic trance may produce a blister on his or her arm when informed that he or she has been burned there, when in fact the subject was touched by an ice cube, or perhaps nothing.

It has been well documented that "mental practice" can improve athletic performance, as for example in basketball: imagining shooting baskets has been shown to translate into measurably more accurate actual shooting.

This list could be extended over several pages, offering instances of how processes we consider mental, or visual, can produce measurable changes in systems we consider bodily or physiological.

Psychoneuroimmunology

Some of the most unsettling---and/or exciting---new findings are about the immune system. As much as any body system, the immune system has been considered autonomous and self-regulating, hardly subject to anything like mental influence.

In 1980, the psychologist, Robert Ader, accidentally discovered that a conditioned suppression could be induced in the immune system of rats. In pursuit of a different research goal, one that need not concern us here, Ader fed his laboratory rats an immuno-suppressive drug flavored with saccharin to make it more palatable. Later, in a kind of serendipitous accident he fed saccharin alone to the rats, and discovered to his surprise that the level of their immune system dropped, as if they had also ingested the drug. Here was a classic Pavlovian conditioned response in the immune system!

The implications here are fascinating and have opened up a whole new arena of research in the interplay of the psychological, neural and immunological networks. The new discipline is called "Psychoneuroimmunology," with a journal and a major text already published.[1]

Question: if the immune system can be depressed by a process (conditioned response) that we have long considered belonged to the realm of the psyche, is it illogical to consider that the immune system might be enhanced by "positive" psychological transactions?

Though we are still shy of hard research documentation of the effectiveness of imagery with cancer and other diseases, it seems very likely that when we find it, it will turn out to be here, in the enhancement of the immune system.

Psychotherapy

Guided imagery has had an important place in the development of modern psychotherapy, beginning in Robert Desoille's "Guided Reverie," and Roberto Assagioli's "Psychosynthesis." Although Freud made little use of it, guided imagery became an important part of Carl Jung's psychology, in a form that he called "Active Imagination." I will return to that later because I have come to believe that my own imagery work closely matches what Jung meant by "Active Imagination."

Even no-nonsense behavior therapists like Joseph Wolpe and Arnold Lazarus make imagery an essential component of their desensitization procedures. In treating, for example, a phobia, the behavior therapist helps his client construct a descriptive "ladder" of feared situations, from least feared to most feared. For example, with a spider phobia, the client might consider least scary the image of a small spider several feet away on the sidewalk. Most scary might be a large hairy spider walking on his face. In between would be eight or ten scenes of graduated scariness. First teaching the client to relax completely, the therapist instructs him to stay in the relaxed state while introducing into his mind's eye the mildest of the frightening images. If the process is designed and monitored properly, the client is able, over time, to move step-by-step up the ladder of imaged scenes, until he/she is able to stay calm and relaxed even while imaging the most feared. The key here is that learned tolerance of imaginary stimuli does translate into tolerance of actual stimuli.

Dean Ornish, M.D., has changed the face of modern cardiology by demonstrating that coronary heart disease can be reversed essentially by changes in life style, diet and exercise. I was fascinated to discover that in his treatment program Ornish also makes use of group psychotherapy, and invites patients to make use of imagery for self-understanding and self-healing. Judging by transcripts of his dialogue with patients in his *Program for Reversing Heart Disease,*[2] Ornish is a gifted psychotherapist and sensitive guide in eliciting healing imagery in his patients.

Active Imagination

Jung is often unclear or inconsistent about some of his basic concepts, and "Active Imagination" is not an exception. Even in other Jungian writers, it has not been easy, at least for me, to find a precise definition of the term. Even harder has been finding a clear procedural guide on how to use it with a client/patient. Perhaps that is as it should be, because if I understand him rightly, Jung is talking about a concept of intrapsychic communication rather than a specific technique for doing it.

Active Imagination consists of a dialogue between the conscious mind and the unconscious, or in Jung's terms, between the Ego and the Self. The Ego asks questions arising from real life problems. Should I marry this woman? Should I change vocations? How can I fight this cancer? And then the Ego listens or watches for an answer. Sometimes the answer may come in a verbal form, but more often it comes in a picture or image, or a series of them. The art is in the listening or watching---how to be open to the answer---because it may come in subtle, strange or unexpected forms.

Both voices in this dialogue between the Ego and the Self are important. If the Ego is absent, as for example in dreaming, then the unconscious sets the agenda as it chooses. On the other hand, if the Ego is too active or forceful in the way it asks, it may limit what it is ready to receive as answers.

I have had some personal experience with that. When I have been very specific in the kind of image I sought as, for example, a warrior to battle cancer cells, I could usually find such an image, but I also found it to lack internal energy and force. I had to keep, as it were, pumping it up. When the image caught me by surprise and seemed to demand a response of some kind from me, it also seemed to carry its own internal energy.

In summary, it is important in Active Imagination, or probably in any form of effective imagery work, for the Ego to ask a significant question, a pointed question, about some aspects of the subject's life, but to ask it in an open-ended way that allows for unanticipated answers.

As a process this is not easy to carry out alone, and most people, myself included, find that it helps to have a helper, a facilitator or guide or listener. The art of guiding is the art of providing enough input to facilitate the inner dialogue of the subject without overguiding, without contaminating or intruding on that inner process. My therapist Jean has a gift for the right balance. When I asked, "Help me figure out how to fight this cancer," she responded in just the right way. She didn't offer me ideas about how she thought I might do that, though she probably had some good ideas. Nor did she overguide by preshaping an image and inviting me to find it. Between us we had the medical information that the site of my cancer activity lay in the bone marrow; so she suggested that I begin an imaginary exploration of my bone marrow to see what I could find. Neither of us had any idea what that would turn out to be; both of us from previous experience had reasons to expect that such a journey might be useful.

Could I have done that work on my own without her? Could I not have suggested to myself that I go exploring in my bone marrow? Perhaps. In one sense I know enough to do that. But it is also true that in spite of how much I know about these processes, my work goes better when I have a good facilitator/guide. I almost said auditor, because sometimes I find that the important role of the facilitator is as listener. I find it important in grasping the imagery to put it into words, to describe it aloud, and when I do that it very much helps to have someone listening, someone who can see the image as I describe it.

Three Voices

So creative imagery work, whether we call it active imagination, visualization, or guided imagery, seems to call for the right balance among three "voices." Two of the voices are within the subject: the Ego and the unconscious. The third voice belongs to the guide, and assists the Ego in forming its questions and in watching for answers.

There are many useful ways for the guide to assist the subject in such imagery, and strategies range from what we could call low profile to high profile. I have found low profile guidance to be more helpful to me; but that fact does not mean that others might not benefit from more active "high profile" guidance. The Simonton's work, for example, as described in their book[3] often has them offering specific images to patients, or inviting the patient's Ego to look for specific images. Their master image for cancer tends to be that of a battle, and therefore they look for and invite the patients to look for warrior images. I have already indicated earlier in this book why I am drawn to images of transforming cancer in preference to "killing" it. But I don't want to discount how useful the Simonton's mode of imagery may be to some patients.

"Interactive Imagery"

I want to recommend strongly another current school of guided imagery that I believe handles the balance among these three "voices" in a truly creative way:

I had the good fortune in April, 1994, to attend in Dallas a two-day training workshop conducted by Martin Rossman and David Bresler, directors of the Academy of Guided Imagery in California.[4] Rossman, a general practice physician, and Bresler, a psychologist, have found guided imagery a valuable tool in their work with patients. Together they have designed, use and teach a down-to-earth, practical group of techniques they have come to call "Interactive Imagery." As the name implies, they see the work as a collaborative enterprise emerging in the dialogue between subject and guide. As guides they offer procedures that I observed, and experienced, as helpful in eliciting resources of the unconscious without over-determining what those resources might be.

One of those processes they call "Meeting Your Inner Advisor." It presupposes that each of us has greater resources of wisdom and knowledge about ourselves, including our bodies, than we normally have conscious access to. If we can invite that inner wisdom to appear in some form of image, it may be able to tell us important things about ourselves that we wouldn't otherwise know. For a full description of this process see Rossman's book.[5]

I want to describe more fully another process they call "Dialogue with the Symptom." Here I summarize and paraphrase a bit, and couch this in the second person, as if inviting the reader to follow along:

Dialogue With the Symptom

1. Begin by getting comfortable. Relax, take a deep breath. As you let it out slowly, let any tension or stress you may feel flow out with it. Let your breathing be deep and regular. Sink into your chair in deeper relaxation. Then as you feel ready . . . . . .

2. Be in a place in your body that needs attention. There may be pain or tension there, or some other sensation asking for your attention.

3. As you are there, or nearing there, allow an image to appear that represents the symptom, or the pain, or the distress in this place.

4. Observe the image. Move closer, examine it carefully, study its features, note its texture, movement, color, temperature, and other characteristics.

5. Notice the feelings you have as you observe.

6. Initiate a dialogue at the feeling level. Ask it what it wants. Does it have something to tell you? Tell it what you may want from it.

7. To go deeper into the feeling, you may want to:

    a. touch the image;

b. become the image.

8. Continue the dialogue until some resolution occurs.

I find it interesting to take this framework back to look at the course of my own imagery journey. In going into my bone marrow, I spontaneously and quite quickly moved through the first five of these stages: relaxing, then going into the bone marrow, seeing an image, reacting emotionally to it, then discovering the shocking fact that these cancer cells were female. The rest of the imagery journey took off from there, but I note that I did not go to Step 6 at that time; I did not try to initiate a dialogue. I think I sensed at the time that these figures were mute, inarticulate and unconscious of what they wanted. Had I asked them I don't think they could have told me.

One can't be sure of something like that, but my hunch is supported by a piece of imagery work done some time later. I was in the Viennese ballroom, enjoying the magic swirl and energy of the dancers. I took occasion politely to interrupt one of the dancing couples, took the young woman aside and asked her what it was like for her before she was brought into the dance,

"Oh," she said, "it was awful, like a nightmare. I was frightened and frantic. I didn't know where I was, or where I was going, or what I was doing."

"Could you have talked to me then if I had asked you to?" I asked.

Her reply: "I don't think so."

Encounter with Nausea

Rossman and Bresler's procedure for "Dialogue with the Symptom" only partly matches the long imagery journey I have already described to you. But I want to add that in their workshop I was able to find something quite useful to me, by engaging in dialogue with a current symptom:

In a practice session with a partner in the workshop who served as my guide, I made a significant discovery about some mild nausea that I had been experiencing recently with my monthly chemotherapy. Since I was a little nauseated at that moment, I was glad for the opportunity, with my partner's help, to do some new exploring.

Going in my imagination down into the area of my stomach, I promptly perceived a kind of dark, oily, turbulent lake, overhung by a black and red sky, with dark clouds and occasional lightning.

"What are you doing here?" I asked.

The oily, heaving lake answered, "I'm just doing my job."

"What is your job?" I asked.

"To get your attention."

"Oh! Well, you certainly have got my attention now. Is there something you want to tell me?"

"Yes. You ought to pay more attention to the fact that when you take chemotherapy every month, you are putting a powerful poison into your body. It kills a lot of cells. You ought to pay more attention to that, learn more about just how chemotherapy acts inside your body. You have been taking all that for granted, not thinking much about it, because your chemotherapy doesn't bother you much. Well, now I'm bothering you---not a lot, but enough to get your attention---because you should pay more attention. I'm not telling you to stop the chemotherapy, just that you shouldn't ignore what it is doing."

My response to all that? "I think you are exactly right. I do believe that I should learn more about that; but in fact I haven't done much study of it. Can you tell me about it?"

Answer: "No, that's not my department. But if you are serious, you know how to look up that information."

My response: "You're right. I'll do that. Thanks for the reminder."

By this time the turbulence in the lake had quieted and my nausea was eased. I thanked my partner for being a good listener/guide.

Driving home from the workshop, I had two additional thoughts:

1. While my imagery work has been emotionally powerful and I believe effective in healing my cancer, it has not included any imagery of what the chemotherapy itself does in my body. I don't have a mental picture of how that poison works. Am I missing something I should go after?

2. That question, then, leads to a deeper awareness: I not only have been vague about how the chemotherapy works in my body, but I have ducked responsibility for it. It has been easy for me to talk about two modes of treatment: what the doctor does and what I do. Imagery, therapy, and so on, are what I do; chemotherapy is what my oncologist does. But as soon as I say it that way, I hear the cop-out. Swallowing chemotherapy pills is in fact what *I* do, not what *h e* does. He prescribes the pills and advises me to take them, and because I trust his advise I follow it. But it is *m y* doing.

If I think it is the right thing for me to do, then I ought to be more than just attentive to it: I ought to get behind it and give it some kind of imaginative push, root for the poison to do its job. I haven't yet found the imagery through which I will do that, but I expect it will appear.

And I still don't know how such imagery will mesh with the "dancing" imagery, which is about transforming cancer cells rather than killing them. But I also expect that I can live with that cognitive dissonance for a while.

NOTES

Chapter One -- My Journey

1. I heard Carl Rogers say this in a seminar at the University of Chicago some forty years ago. If it appears in his writings, I have not found it.

2. O. Carl Simonton, Stephanie-Matthews Simonton, and James Creighton, **Getting Well Again.** New York: Bantam Books, 1978.

3. One valuable source is the International Myeloma Foundation, 2120 Stanley Hills Drive, Los Angeles, CA 90046. They publish a quarterly newsletter on research and treatment of myeloma.

4. **Wintrobe's Clinical Hematology,** Ninth Edition, Vol. 2, Chapter 84. Philadelphia: Lea and Febiger, 1993.

5. Cornelius Beaukencamp wrote **Fortunate Strangers,** now out of print, one of the earliest accounts of group therapy.

6. Joseph Zinker, **The Creative Process in Gestalt Therapy.** New York: Vintage, 1978.

7. Harville Hendrix, **Getting the Love You Want.** New York: Henry Holt, 1988. See this book for an engaging discussion of how we are likely to select unconsciously as a partner someone with whom we can re-enact unfinished issues from childhood.

8. David J. Grove and B. I. Panzer, **Resolving Traumatic Memories.** New York: Irvington Publishers, 1991.

9. Robert Bly, **Iron John: A Book About Men.** New York: Addison Wesley, 1990.

10. Jeanne Achterberg, **Imagery In Healing: Shamanism and Modern Medicine.** Boston: Shambhala, 1985.

   ----- and Frank Lawlis, **Imagery of Cancer.** Champaign, Illinois: Institute for Personality and Ability Testing, 1978.

-----and Frank Lawlis, *Bridges of the Body-Mind: Behavioral Approaches to Health Care.* Champaign, Illinois: Institute for Personality and Ability Testing, 1980.

-----Barbara Dossey and Leslie Kolkmeier, *Rituals of Healing.* New York: Bantam, 1994.

Frank Lawlis, *The Cure: The Hero's Journey With Cancer.* San Jose, CA: Resource Publications, 1994.

11. Bruce Chatwin, *Songlines.* New York: Viking, 1987.

12. See for example: Walter Truitt Anderson, *Reality Isn't What It Used To Be.* Harper San Francisco, 1990.

Chapter Two -- Reflections

1. *Wintrobe's Clinical Hematology.* Ninth Edition, Vol. 2, Chapter 84. Philadelphia: Lea and Febiger, 1993.

2. Bill Moyers, *Healing and the Mind.* New York: Doubleday, 1993.

3. Norman Cousins, *Anatomy of an Illness.* New York: Norton, 1979.

4. O. Carl Simonton, Stephanie-Matthews Simonton, and James Creighton, *Getting Well Again.* New York: Bantam Books, 1978.

Chapter Four -- Where's Brute Now?

1. Anatole Broyard, *Intoxicated by My Illness.* New York: Clarkson Potter Publishers, 1992. Page 7.

2. Shaffer calls his model "Transformational Fantasy." It has been made the centerpiece of the "GETTING WELL" behavioral medicine program in Orlando, Florida. The director of that program, Dierdre Davis Brigham, has written about her program and about Transformational Fantasy in her book, *Imagery for Getting Well* (New York: Norton, 1994).

Chapter Five -- Thoughts About Life and Death

1. Anatole Broyard, *Intoxicated by My Illness.* New York: Clarkson Potter Publishers, 1992. Page 23.

2. Brendan O'Regan and Caryle Hirshberg, *Spontaneous Remissions: An Annotated Bibliography.* Sausalito, California: Institute for Noetic Sciences, 1993.

3. Bernie Siegel, *Love, Medicine and Miracles.* New York: Harper and Row, 1986.

   —— *Peace, Love and Healing.* New York: Harper and Row, 1989.

   —— *How to Live Between Office Visits.* New York: Harper Collins, 1993.

4. Larry Dossey, *Space, Time and Medicine.* Boston: Shambhala, 1982.

   ——*Beyond Illness.* Boston: Shambhala, 1984.

   ——*Recovering the Soul.* Bantam Books, 1989.

   ——*Meaning and Medicine.* New York: Bantam Books, 1991.

5. Deepak Chopra, *Unconditional Life.* New York: Bantam Books, 1991. Page 24.

6. Ken Wilber, *Grace and Grit.* Boston: Shambhala, 1991.

7. Ken Wilber, *The Holographic Paradigm.* Boston: Shambhala,1982.

   ——*Up From Eden: A Transpersonal View of Evolution.* Anchor, 1981.

   ——*No Boundary: Eastern and Western Approaches to Personal Growth.* Boston: Shambhala, 1979.

8. *Grace and Grit,* pages 338-9.

9. Sherwin B. Nuland, *How We Die: Reflections on Life's Final Chapter.* New York: Alfred A. Knopf, 1994.

Appendix A -- Complementary Treatments for Cancer

1. Paul Trachtman, "NIH Looks at the Implausible and the Inexplicable." *The Smithsonian,* September 1992.

2. *The Cancer Chronicles,* March, 1994. Otho, Iowa: Equinox Press.

3. Michael Lerner, *Choices In Healing: Integrating the Best of Conventional and Complementary Approaches to Cancer.* Boston, M.I.T. Press, 1994.

4. Bill Moyers, *Healing and the Mind.* New York: Doubleday, 1993.

5. Raymond H. Murray, M.D., and Arthur J. Rubel, Ph.D., *New England Journal of Medicine,* January 2, 1992.

6. University of Texas at Dallas.

7. Quoted in Lerner, Op.Cit., page 176.

8. Lawrence LeShan, *Cancer as a Turning Point.* New York: Penguin Plume Books, 1989.

9. Ibid., page 7.

10. Ibid, pages 8-10.

11. Lawrence LeShan, *You Can Fight for Your Life: Emotional Factors In the Treatment of Cancer.* New York: Evans, 1979.

12. W. H. Auden, *Collected Shorter Poems 1927-1957.* New York: Random House, 1966.

13. Susan Sontag, *Illness As Metaphor.* New York: Farrar, Strauss and Giroux, 1977.

14. Lerner (see Note #3), page 178.

15. Henry Dreher, *Your Defense Against Cancer.* New York: Harper Paperbooks, 1994, page 332.

16. Dreher, pages 342-345.

17. Lydia Temoshok and Henry Dreher, *The Type C Connection: The Mind-Body Link to Cancer and Your Health.* New York: Penguin Plume Books, 1993.

18. Dreher, page 347.

19. Lerner (see Note #3), page 154.

20. Lerner (see Note #3), page 159.

21. Paul Wilkes, *In Mysterious Ways: The Life and Death of a Parish Priest.* New York: Avon, 1990.

22. Lawrence LeShan, *You Can Fight For Your Life.* New York: Evans, 1979.

    ----*Cancer As a Turning Point.* New York: Dutton, 1989.

23. Lawrence LeShan, "Mobilizing the Life Force," audio tape available from Sounds True Recordings, 735 Walnut St., Boulder, CO80302.

Appendix B -- Visualization

1. Robert Ader, David L. Felton, and Nicholas Cohen, eds., *Psychoneuroimmunology,* Second Edition. San Diego: Academic Press, 1991.

2. Dean Ornish, *Program for Reversing Heart Disease.* New York: Ballantine Books, 1990.

3. O. Carl Simonton, Stephanie-Matthews Simonton, and James Creighton, *Getting Well Again.* New York: Bantam Books, 1978.

4. Academy of Guided Imagery, P.O.Box 2070, Mill Valley, CA 94942.

5. Martin Rossman, *Healing Yourself.* New York: Pocket Books, 1989. Chapter 7.

About the Author

Robert E. Elliott grew up in Tacoma, Washington, where he was graduated from the College (now University) of Puget Sound. In World War II he served as pilot of a four-engined B-24 bomber, flying thirty-five missions out of Italy, and was awarded the Distinguished Flying Cross.

After the war he took a degree in divinity from Yale University, and led Methodist congregations in Seattle and Chicago. From the University of Chicago he received the degree of Ph.D. in Religion and Personality. In 1955 he joined the faculty of the Perkins School of Theology, Southern Methodist University, in Dallas, Texas. After twenty-four years of teaching counseling and psychology, he resigned his position to enter full-time clinical practice.

In that private practice he has been closely associated with his friend and former teaching colleague, Harville Hendrix, creator of "Imago Relationship Therapy," author of *Getting the Love You Want* and other important books on primary relationships. Dr. Elliott currently serves as the Director of the Center for (Imago) Relationship Therapy in Dallas, where he conducts "Getting the Love You Want" workshops for couples.

He is a licensed supervisor of marriage and family therapists in the state of Texas, an Approved Supervisor in the American Association for Marriage and Family Therapy, and a Diplomate in the American Association of Pastoral Counselors.

Other professional memberships include: Association for Imago Relationship Therapy, Dallas Association for Marriage and Family Therapy (past president), American Group Psychotherapy Association, Southwest Group Psychotherapy Association, Dallas Group Psychotherapy Society, and North Texas Society for Clinical Hypnosis.

He serves as Designated Counselor to clergy families in the North Texas Conference of the United Methodist Church, and holds retired clergy status in that Conference.

In 1994, he has begun to broaden the scope of his psychotherapy practice to include work with cancer patients.

His wife, Dorothy Gail Elliott, is a music educator and writer. They have three grown children and two grandchildren.

* *

ADDENDUM (June, 1997)

My husband, Dr. Robert Elliott, died on March 21, 1997, of multiple myeloma, the cancer finally depleting his immune system so he could not recover from infections.

On January 6 Bob had come down with his third case of severe bronchitis in eight months, and was again hospitalized. Antibiotics overcame the bronchitis, but acute colitis developed which left him very weak. When two rounds of chemotherapy failed to bring positive results, he was allowed to come home on March 1. I cared for him, then, for his last three weeks---with the help of Hospice nurses.

Bob was glad to be home, but he hated to be of "bother" to me. He had been in "control" of his multiple myeloma for so many years that he found it hard to accept the fact that it now controlled him. However, he accepted his approaching death with grace and dignity. While still in the hospital, he talked about how he felt: that he had had a good life; that he was at a good stopping place; that he didn't even have any clients in crisis at that time. He actually counselled quite effectively two clients in his hospital room, and that work meant a great deal to him as well as to them. One of his long-running therapy groups came to his bedside for a "goodbye" session with him. Another, Group 17---the therapy group to which he belonged for so many years---came to the house the week before he died to extend their support and love to him and to me, and to tell Bob what he had meant to each of them.. Bob loved them so much, and they him.

One of Bob's professional friends, who had been an almost daily visitor those last weeks, arranged for Bob to receive his war-time medals that had never caught up with him. Our Congressional representative came to the house to present them, bringing with him the press and TV. Then a few days before Bob's death, the DALLAS MORNING NEWS ran a beautiful story about the event and a little about Bob's life, complete with a full-color picture of Bob taken as our son John leaned over to kiss him on the forehead after the ceremony. Friends gave us a video copy of Channel 5's newscast of the event, and we all watched that many times---Bob seeming to be somewhat embarrassed about all the "fuss" everyone was making over him and his war-time achievements.

Numerous personal friends, ex-students and profess-ional friends came to his bedside to express their appreciation for his work with them. The cards and letters poured in, many with testimonials of Bob's work with them. I went through these after Bob's death, typing out two pages of excerpts of the most moving; son Bruce read these at the memorial service as a preface to inviting people to speak about Bob. A dozen or more responded, and it was very heart-warming.

You may want to turn to page 88 in this book and read what Bob had to say about dying and the prospects of his own death. He certainly did "relinquish life gracefully and gratefully" when his time came. But it was hard for friends and family to let him go. We were certainly grateful for his life, and did not want him to suffer longer; but we knew how sorely we would miss him.

The hole in this survivor's heart is huge and aching. But I remember the almost fifty years we have had together, and am beginning to realize what a fortunate woman I have been!

Dorothy G. Elliott

Additional copies of this book
may be ordered from:

NOTEMAN PRESS

2603 Andrea Lane
Dallas, TX 75228

214/327-4466

ORDER FORM

	No. of copies	Total
Dancing With Cancer @ $ 11.95	_____	$_____
Mailing and handling: $1.50; add 50 ¢ each additional book.		$_____
Texas residents add 99¢ sales tax per copy.		$_____
Grand Total		$_____

Make check payable to NOTEMAN PRESS. Credit cards not accepted.

Send to:
